FOGSI EEBR 2025

Ethical Evidence-Based Recommendations

Genetics in Obstetrics and Gynecology

Disclaimer

This Ethical Evidence-Based Recommendation (EEBR) document is drafted following a consensus between esteemed FOGSI experts and stakeholders and are based on the scientific evidence available at the time of preparation.

EEBRs should be used for information and educational purposes. They do not replace the need for application of clinical judgment to each individual presentation, or variations based on individual patient and resource setting.

Furthermore, EEBRs do not constitute or imply the endorsement of any of the included technologies, therapies, or techniques by FOGSI.

FOGSI EEBR 2025

Ethical Evidence-Based Recommendations

Genetics in Obstetrics and Gynecology

Editor-in-Chief

Sunita Tandulwadkar

MD (Obs and Gyne) FICS (Gyne-Endoscopy) FICOG
President, FOGSI (2025–2026)
Gynecological Endoscopist and ART & IVF Specialist
Head, Department of Obstetrics and Gynecology
Chief, IVF & Endoscopy Center, Ruby Hall Clinic, Pune
Founder and Medical Director
Solo Clinic IVF—A Center for Excellence in Infertility and Endoscopy, Pune
Founder and Medical Director
Solo Stem Cells—A Stem Cell Research and Application Center, Pune
Founder and Director, Alive Regenerative Wellness, Pune, Maharashtra, India

Editor

Vandana Bansal

MBBS MD DGO DNB FICOG FRCOG (UK) FNB (High Risk Pregnancy and Perinatology)
Additional Professor and Head of Ultrasound
Department of Obstetrics and Gynecology
and Fetal Medicine
Nowrosjee Wadia Maternity Hospital and
Seth GS Medical College
Mumbai, Maharashtra, India

Expert

Mandakini Pradhan

MD DNB DM (Medical Genetics)
Professor and Head
Department of Maternal and Reproductive Health
Sanjay Gandhi Post Graduate Institute of Medical Sciences
Lucknow, Uttar Pradesh, India

Convener

Pooja Lodha

DNB (Obs and Gyne)
Fellow, Fetal Medicine, FOGSI-FMF UK Certified
Lead Consultant
Department of Fetal Medicine
Ruby Hall Clinic and Bharati Vidyapeeth University and Hospital, Pune
Director, Kangaroo Cradle, Fetal Care Centre
Pune, Maharashtra, India

JAYPEE BROTHERS MEDICAL PUBLISHERS

The Health Sciences Publisher

New Delhi | London

Jaypee Brothers Medical Publishers (P) Ltd

Headquarters
Jaypee Brothers Medical Publishers (P) Ltd
EMCA House, 23/23-B
Ansari Road, Daryaganj
New Delhi 110 002, India
Landline: +91-11-23272143, +91-11-23272703
+91-11-23282021, +91-11-23245672
Email: jaypee@jaypeebrothers.com

Corporate Office
Jaypee Brothers Medical Publishers (P) Ltd
4838/24, Ansari Road, Daryaganj
New Delhi 110 002, India
Phone: +91-11-43574357
Fax: +91-11-43574314
Email: jaypee@jaypeebrothers.com

Overseas Office
JP Medical Ltd.
83, Victoria Street, London
SW1H 0HW (UK)
Phone: +44 20 3170 8910
Fax: +44 (0)20 3008 6180
Email: info@jpmedpub.com

Website: www.jaypeebrothers.com
Website: www.jaypeedigital.com

Inquiries for bulk sales may be solicited at: jaypee@jaypeebrothers.com

FOGSI EEBR 2025—Ethical Evidence-Based Recommendations: Genetics in Obstetrics and Gynecology

First Edition: **2025**

ISBN: 978-93-6616-693-3

Printed in India

Contributors

Angela Devanboo
MSc (Med Sci) in Medical Genetics
Lead Genome Analyst
Department of NIPT
MedGenome Labs Ltd.
Bengaluru, Karnataka, India

Asmita Thakur
MSc (Genetic Engineering)
Intern
Department of Genetics and
Molecular Medicine
Kokilaben Dhirubhai Ambani Hospital
and Medical Research Institute
Mumbai, Maharashtra, India

Bibhas Kar
PhD (Life Science)
Consultant and Head
Department of Genetics and
Molecular Medicine
Kokilaben Dhirubhai Ambani Hospital
and Medical Research Institute
Mumbai, Maharashtra, India

Chaitanya A Datar
MBBS MD (Medical Genetics)
Director, Sujanan Clinics, Pune
Consultant
Genetics Unit
Department of Pediatrics
Bharati Hospital and Research Center
Pune, Maharashtra, India

Hema Purandarey
MBBS MS FICMH PhD (Genetics)
Consultant and Medical Director
(Prenatal and Reproductive Geneticist)
MedGenome Centre for Genetic
Healthcare
Mumbai, Maharashtra, India

Juili Bharankar MSc
Technical Assistant (Project)
Department of Genetic Research Centre
ICMR—National Institute for Research
in Reproductive and Child Health
Mumbai, Maharashtra, India

Keshav Malhotra
MBBS MCE ESHRE Certified
Clinical Embryologist
Lab Director, ART Rainbow IVF
Agra, Uttar Pradesh, India
Vice Chairman, Embryology ISAR
Chairman, Embryology SIG ASPIRE
Executive Committee Member, Alpha
Scientists, ACE, ISPAT

Mandakini Pradhan
MD DNB DM (Medical Genetics)
Professor and Head
Department of Maternal and
Reproductive Health
Sanjay Gandhi Post Graduate
Institute of Medical Sciences
Lucknow, Uttar Pradesh, India

Niharika Jadeja
MMSc (Human Genetics and
Genetic Counseling)
Genetic Counselor
Department of Clinical Genetics
The Purple Gene Clinic
Mumbai, Maharashtra, India

Palak Sharma MBBS
DY Patil University School of Medicine
Mumbai, Maharashtra, India

Parag M Tamhankar
DM (Medical Genetics) MD DNB
DCH FCPS (Pediatrics)
Consultant Medical Geneticist
Centre for Medical Genetics
Mumbai, Maharashtra, India

Prakash Gambhir MD
Chief Medical Scientist
LifeCell Diagnostics, Pune
Director, Birthright Genetic Clinic
Pune, Maharashtra, India

Pratiksha Chheda
PhD (Biotechnology)
Lead Molecular Biologist
Department of Molecular Diagnostics
Sir HN Reliance Foundation Hospital
and Research Centre
Mumbai, Maharashtra, India

Priya Kadam MBBS MS (Genetics)
Director Reproductive Genomics
Department of Operations
MedGenome Labs Ltd.
Bengaluru, Karnataka, India

Rajiv Sarin
MD FRCR (Clinical Oncology)
In-Charge, Cancer Genetics Unit
Department of Cancer Genetics
Tata Memorial Hospital and ACTREC
Mumbai, Maharashtra, India

Ratna Dua Puri
MD DM (Medical Genetics)
Head
Department of Genetics
Institute of Medical Genetics
and Genomics
Sir Ganga Ram Hospital
New Delhi, India

Rupal Parekh Tulle
MBBS DNB (Obs and Gyne)
DGO (Gold Medalist)
Consultant
Department of Fetal Medicine
Borneo Mother and Child Hospital
Thane West, Maharashtra, India

Shagun Aggarwal
MD DM ECMGG Certified
Professor
Department of Medical Genetics
Nizam's Institute of Medical Sciences
Hyderabad, Telangana, India

Sailesh Pande MBBS MS FDBT (Fellow)
Scientist E and Head
Department of Genetic
Research Centre
ICMR—National Institute for Research
in Reproductive and Child Health
Mumbai, Maharashtra, India

Shalin S Vaniawala MBBS
Medical Officer
SN Gene Lab Pvt Ltd
Surat, Gujarat, India

Shruti Bajaj
MD Pediatrics (MUHS) Fellowship in
Clinical Genetics (MUHS) Masters in
Neurometabolism and Cell Biology
(University of Barcelona, Spain)
Director and Consultant
Department of Clinical Genetics
The Purple Gene Clinic
Mumbai, Maharashtra, India

Sunita Tandulwadkar
MD (Obs and Gyne) FICS (Gyne-Endoscopy)
FICOG
President, FOGSI (2025–2026)
Gynecological Endoscopist and
ART & IVF Specialist
Head, Department of Obstetrics and
Gynecology
Chief, IVF & Endoscopy Center
Ruby Hall Clinic, Pune
Founder and Medical Director
Solo Clinic IVF—A Center for Excellence
in Infertility and Endoscopy, Pune
Founder and Medical Director
Solo Stem Cells—A Stem Cell Research
and Application Center, Pune
Founder and Director
Alive Regenerative Wellness
Pune, Maharashtra, India

Tasneem Shaikh
MSc (Genetic Counseling)
Genetic Counselor
Department of Clinical Genetics
The Purple Gene Clinic
Mumbai, Maharashtra, India

Usha Dave MSc PhD DHA
Laboratory Director
Scientific and Technical Operations and Research Director
Department of Metabolic and Molecular Genetics
Clinical and Laboratory Diagnosis
INavigene Genetic Science Lab and MILS International India
Mumbai, Maharashtra, India

Vandana Bansal
MBBS MD DGO DNB FICOG FRCOG (UK) FNB (High Risk Pregnancy and Perinatology)
Additional Professor and Head of Ultrasound
Department of Obstetrics and Gynecology and Fetal Medicine
Nowrosjee Wadia Maternity Hospital and Seth GS Medical College
Mumbai, Maharashtra, India

Vandana Chaddha
MS (Obs and Gyne) Clinical Fellow Maternal-Fetal Medicine (University of Toronto)
Consultant
Department of Fetal Medicine
Sattva the Fetal Medicine Centre
New Delhi, India

Vasundhara P Tamhankar
DNB DCH (Pediatrics) Fellowship in Genetics (DHR)
Consultant Medical Geneticist and Pediatrician
Centre for Medical Genetics
Mumbai, Maharashtra, India

Preface

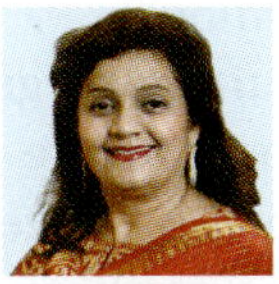

Editor-in-Chief
Sunita Tandulwadkar

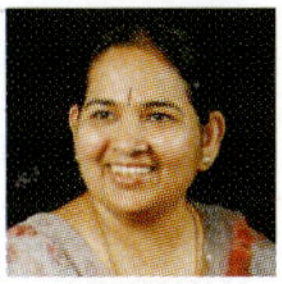

Editor
Vandana Bansal

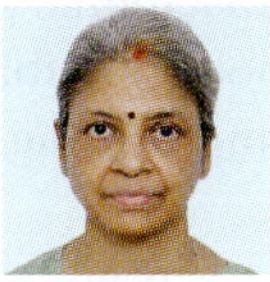

Expert
Mandakini Pradhan

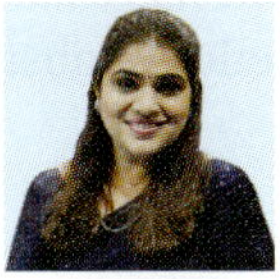

Convener
Pooja Lodha

In our pursuit of advancing women's health in India, establishing our own ethical evidence-based recommendations is essential. As the President of the Federation of Obstetric and Gynaecological Societies of India (FOGSI) 2025, I am delighted to present this *Ethical Evidence-Based Recommendations on Genetics in Obstetrics and Gynecology*, a comprehensive resource developed with insights from leading experts across the country. While international organizations such as the International Federation of Gynecology and Obstetrics (FIGO), American Society for Reproductive Medicine (ASRM), European Society of Human Reproduction and Embryology (ESHRE), and Royal College of Obstetricians and Gynaecologists (RCOG) have established detailed recommendations, India has yet to create a unified, evidence-based framework in this area. This publication aims to bridge that gap, providing Indian practitioners with accessible, thorough recommendations for integrating genetics into obstetrics and gynecology care.

Understanding genetics is pivotal to modern obstetric and gynecological practice, with profound implications for prenatal, perinatal, and reproductive care. These ethical evidence-based recommendations begin with foundational concepts in medical genetics, equipping practitioners with essential knowledge for navigating complex genetic information. Following this, pedigree charting is introduced as a critical tool for assessing inherited risks, guiding practitioners in creating detailed family histories to better understand genetic inheritance patterns.

The publication also provides guidance on carrier screening and genetic inheritance, highlighting key strategies for identifying and managing inherited conditions. Preconception genetic counseling is covered in depth, offering protocols to help practitioners provide essential genetic insights into couples planning a pregnancy. Further, prenatal screening options, diagnostic testing, and noninvasive prenatal testing (NIPT) are presented with evidence-backed guidelines, ensuring safe, accurate screening and diagnostics for early detection.

Recommendations on managing common congenital anomalies and their genetic associations follow, alongside a section on fetal autopsy and placental pathology, which provide valuable protocols for understanding fetal anomalies and losses. A targeted chapter addresses approaches to intellectual disabilities, both with and without dysmorphism, offering practitioners insights into prenatal diagnosis for these conditions.

Additional recommendations cover the genetics of recurrent pregnancy loss, aiding practitioners in identifying genetic causes to provide more informed, compassionate care. The publication also details the genetic management of hemoglobinopathies and introduces the application of molecular technology in prenatal diagnosis, ensuring that practitioners are equipped with the latest advances in genetic technology.

Finally, a dedicated section on research advances and future directions in obstetric genetics provides a forward-looking view, preparing practitioners to adapt to emerging trends in genetics and precision medicine in the field.

This publication represents FOGSI's commitment to equipping Indian gynecologists with the latest scientific advancements, framed within our cultural and clinical context. I am deeply grateful to the multidisciplinary team whose collaborative efforts have made these recommendations possible. We hope they become a trusted companion for practitioners, empowering them to deliver compassionate, evidence-based care in genetics.

Through this initiative, FOGSI reaffirms its dedication to advancing women's health and setting a new standard for ethical, informed care. We trust that these ethical evidence-based recommendations will serve as both a valuable guide and an inspiration for the integration of genetics in obstetrics and gynecology across India.

Contents

CHAPTER 1

Conventional Genetics and Cytogenomics

Sailesh Pande, Juili Bharankar

Q1. What is Karyotyping?

Karyotyping involves study of chromosome i.e., identifying and sorting chromosomes according to their banding pattern. It is a widely used technique to detect alterations in chromosome. Chromosomes are classified according to their length, band pattern, and position of centromere. It can detect numerical and structural chromosomal abnormalities.

Q2. What are different types of chromosomes?

Based on the position of centromere there are four types of chromosomes—Metacentric, sub-metacentric, acrocentric, and telocentric. There are two arms, one above the centromere is p arm and one below centromere is q arm.

i. *Metacentric chromosomes:* Chromosome in which the centromere is located in the center results in both the p arm and q arm being of equal length is called a metacentric chromosome. In humans, chromosome 1, 3, 16, 19, and 20 are metacentric chromosomes.
ii. *Sub-metacentric chromosomes:* Chromosomes in which the centromere is slightly-off center, this results in the longer q arm and comparatively shorter p arm are sub-metacentric chromosomes. In humans, chromosome 2, 4, 5, 6 to 12, 17, 18 and X are sub metacentric chromosomes.
iii. *Acrocentric chromosomes:* Chromosomes in which the centromere is located near one end, these results in a very short p arm and very long q arm are acrocentric chromosomes. In humans, chromosome 13, 14, 15, 21, 22 and Y are acrocentric chromosomes.
iv. *Telocentric chromosomes:* In this chromosome, centromere is located at the end, this results in only one long q arm. Telocentric chromosomes are not present in humans.

Q3. What are different tissues on which cytogenetic test can be performed?

Draft recommendations and evidence: Cytogenetic tests can be performed on the different types of tissues depending on the clinical requirement and the type of data required. The most common type of the tissues used in cytogenetic tests are: Peripheral blood, amniotic fluid, chorionic villi, products of conception including fetal skin and rarely from bone marrow. However there is a 50% chance of culture failure in an abortus sample.

Q4. What are different types of cytogenetic staining and Banding methods?

Draft recommendations and evidence: Different types of cytogenetic staining and banding methods are:

i. *G Banding:* In this technique, chromosomes are stained by Giemsa dye after trypsin treatment. This technique produces a characteristic banding pattern of light and dark bands.

ii. *R. Banding:* R banding also called as reverse banding. Here banding pattern is reverse of G-Band.

iii. *Q-Banding:* In this technique, the chromosomes are stained by using a fluorescent dye called quinacrine that binds to specific chromatin regions.

iv. *C-Banding:* In this technique chromosomes are treated to stain the centromeric region of the chromosome.

v. *AgNOR:* It is silver staining (AgNOR) for nucleolus organizing regions. Nucleolus organizing regions (NORs) are the segments of the chromosome that consists of the ribosomal genes which are necessary for the synthesis of 18S and 28S rRNA in humans. NORs when silver stained are called as AgNORs. AgNOR appears as the well-defined black dots under the light microscope after silver staining. It reveals acrocentric chromosomal rearrangements and polymorphisms.

Q5. What are applications of karyotyping in obstetrics and gynecological practice?

Draft recommendations and evidence:

- *Recurrent pregnancy losses:* Couple with recurrent pregnancy loss can have balanced translocation of chromosome. The balanced translocation may be reciprocal (between two chromosomes) or Robertsonian (between two acrocentric chromosomes). Apart from translocation, it can be inversion (para- or pericentric inversion) or unbalanced like deletion or duplication. Genetic testing of products of conception (POCs) provides essential information for reproductive counseling.
- *In pubertal disorders:* Karyotyping as a basic genetic test plays important role in pubertal disorders such as menstrual abnormalities, uterine and ovarian abnormalities, gynecomastia, hypogonadism etc.
- *Infertility testing:* Infertile couple can have chromosomal abnormalities especially male infertility. Female with anovulation can have mosaicism for sex chromosome and hence chromosomal analysis of couple is suggested before undergoing IVF.
- *In prenatal diagnosis:* Fetus identified to be at high risk for aneuploidy after combined screening, identification of malformation on ultrasound associated with high risk for chromosomal abnormality are to be subjected for prenatal diagnosis for chromosomal abnormality. If found normal

then further testing like chromosomal microarray and exome sequencing may be warranted.

- *In mental sub-normality:* Karyotyping should be the first step of genetic test in mental sub-normality.

Q6. What are different types of chromosomal abnormalities seen in recurrent pregnancy loss, infertility and pubertal disorders?

Draft recommendations and evidence:

- *Recurrent pregnancy loss:* Balanced translocations or inversion etc.
- *Infertility:* Sex chromosomal abnormalities
- *Pubertal disorders:* Turner's Syndrome in female and Klinefelter's syndrome in male. Rarely it can be other sex chromosome abnormality like 47, XXX, 47, XXY.

Q7. What are different types of chromosomal abnormalities and patterns seen in Down syndrome, Turner syndrome, Patau syndrome?

Draft recommendations and evidence:

Down syndrome: Down syndrome is caused due to an additional copy of chromosome 21. This results in the three copies of chromosome 21 instead of normal two. There are primarily 3 patterns seen in Down syndrome

i. *Free trisomy 21:* It consists of an extra copy of chromosome 21 in every cell and hence total chromosome number will be 47 in every cell.
ii. *Mosaic trisomy 21:* It consists of two distinct cell lines, one with the normal number of chromosomes and another with the additional copy of chromosome 21.
iii. *Robertsonian translocation:* In this type, the entire long arm of chromosome 21 is attached to another chromosome, typically an acrocentric chromosome like 13, 14, 21 or 22.

Turner syndrome: Turner syndrome is the condition characterized by the complete or the partial loss of one of the two sex chromosomes. This results in Monosomy X. Patterns seen in Turner syndrome:

i. *Monosomy X:* It consists of only one copy of chromosome X instead of two.
ii. *Mosaic turner:* It consists of mosaic pattern of cells, meaning it consists of two different cell lines one 45, X and another 46, XX/XY.
iii. *Isochromosome Xq:* It consists of the replication of the long arm of X chromosome.
iv. *Ring chromosome X:* X chromosome forms a ring structure. This can lead to the complete or partial inactivation of X chromosome.

Patau syndrome: Trisomy 13, also known as Patau syndrome, is named after Dr. Patau, the scientist who discovered and genetically categorized the syndrome. This chromosomal disorder is caused by the presence of an extra copy of chromosome 13. Different patterns seen in Patau syndrome are:

i. *Complete Trisomy 13 or Full Trisomy:* This condition is characterized by having the three copies of Chromosome 13 in all the cells. This condition is also called as simple trisomy 13 or free trisomy 13.
ii. *Mosaic Trisomy 13:* This is the condition in which only some cells of the body will have three copies of chromosome 13 while other cells will have normal two copies of chromosome 13.
iii. *Partial Trisomy 13:* This is a rare condition in which only a portion of the chromosome 13 is present in the triplicate in each cell.
iv. *Robertsonian translocation 13:* It is a condition which is characterized by having two standard copies of chromosome 13 and an extra copy of chromosome 13 which is translocated to another chromosome usually they are acrocentric chromosomes.

Q8. What is fluorescence in situ hybridization (FISH)?

Draft recommendations and evidence: Fluorescence in situ hybridization (FISH) is a technique for identifying specific and targeted DNA sequences. This technique involves using fluorescently labeled DNA or RNA probes that bind to specific target sequences in the sample DNA, which can be further visualized under fluorescent microscope. It can detect presence or absence the chromosome or part of the chromosome for which the specific probe was used. Example: If probe for chromosome 21 is used and there are 3 fluorescence signals detected then it's interpreted as 3 copies of chromosome 21 or Trisomy 21 or Down syndrome. Hence, FISH test is ordered for the specific disease that is suspected on clinical examination. It is also used to diagnose genetic disorders, gene mapping, and find novel oncogenes or genetic anomalies linked to certain cancers.

Q9. What are different types of FISH and their utility in clinical practice?

Draft recommendations and evidence:

- *Interphase FISH:* Interphase Fluorescence in Situ Hybridization (IFISH), involves use of probes that are labeled with fluorochromes to detect chromosomal abnormalities within the intact nuclei. Interphase FISH is performed on blood, abortus material, bone marrow and can also be performed on the tissue sections that are paraffin-embedded and formalin-fixed.

  Utility: It is used in the identification of numerical chromosomal disorders (13, 18, 21, 16, 22 X and Y) in POCs and in prenatal diagnosis. It is a valuable cytogenetic method in investigating chromosome abnormalities in cancer. It is also well-established method for diagnosing and evaluating hematolymphoid malignancies and low grade mosaicism in syndromes such as Downs, Turners, and Klinefelter.

- *Metaphase FISH:* Metaphase FISH resulted in strong and specific fluorescent staining of human chromosomes in metaphase spreads.
- *Utility:* It is used in identification of various microdeletions syndromes, solid tumors and hematolymphoid malignancies for detecting abnormalities like deletions/duplications, amplification, translocations.
- *Whole chromosome paint:* Whole chromosome paint uses fluorescent labeled DNA probes to create a "paint" that homogenously stains the entire chromosome in one color. Different chromosomes can have different color and hence origin of a marker chromosome or a ring chromosome can be identified.

  Utility: Used in detection of unbalanced translocations, identification of marker chromosome.

Q10. What are the limitations of FISH and karyotyping?

Draft recommendations and evidence:

Limitations of FISH:

i. This technique is limited to evaluating few anomalies at a time and is capable of detecting the abnormalities that can be detected by using the current probes available. It cannot detect abnormalities if the probes for that specific region are not available.
ii. It is used for detecting specific target region on the chromosome; this makes FISH less effective screening technique for disease with cytogenetic diversity.
iii. FISH is highly sensitive for detecting trisomy and it is less effective for identifying chromosome loss or deletions.
iv. Processing bone marrow or peripheral blood samples for FISH is comparatively easy, but preparing paraffin-embedded tissues or frozen sections from solid tumors or lymph node biopsies for FISH is considerably more complex.

Limitations of karyotyping:

i. Karyotyping technique has low resolution as compared to other genetic techniques.
ii. Karyotype is limited technique due to its inability to detect the complex abnormalities, cryptic aberration and marker chromosome accurately.
iii. Due to its low resolution this technique cannot detect, microdeletions and micro-duplications.
iv. This technique needs viable cells only. It cannot be performed on nonviable cells, nonviable tissue, or macerated, tissue.
v. Maintenance of cell culture and processing can be challenging task. Lack of good metaphase, less or no metaphase in slide, poor bands, clumped chromosomes, overlapping chromosomes etc., are the various challenges faced in karyotyping techniques.

Q11. What is Mendelian inheritance?

Scientist Gregor Mendel studied characteristics in pea plants, including flower color, pea color, and pea shape. Through these studies he established the principles of segregation, independent assortment, and dominance. The traits Mendel studied were controlled by single genes, each had two alternative alleles, one dominant and one recessive, this determined the phenotypes.

It applies to disease due to an alteration in a single gene. The gene may be located on autosome or on sex chromosome. Depending on the type of inheritance it can be recessive (manifestation when both the copies are abnormal) or dominant (manifestation even on copy is abnormal).

BIBLIOGRAPHY

1. Alkhamessi RN, Al-Bayaty MK, Ibraheem HT. Patau syndrome, prevalence and natural history. Sci Res Jr Med Sci. 2023;3(1):5-9.
2. Arsham MS, Barch MJ, Lawce HJ. The AGT Cytogenetics Laboratory Manual, 4th edition. New Jersey, United States: Wiley-Blackwell; 2017.
3. Berisha SZ, Shetty S, Prior TW, et al. Cytogenetic and molecular diagnostic testing associated with prenatal and postnatal birth defects. Birth Defects Res. 2020;112(4):293-306.
4. Bhat TA, Wani AA. Fluorescence in situ hybridization (FISH) and its applications. Chromosome Structure and Aberrations. 2017:343-67.
5. Liu Y, Sun XC, Lv GJ, et al. Amniotic fluid karyotype analysis and prenatal diagnosis strategy of 3117 pregnant women with amniocentesis indication. J Comp Eff Res. 2023;12(6):e220168.
6. McGowan-Jordan J, Hastings RJ, Moore S. ISCN 2020: An International system for human cytogenomic nomenclature. Basel: Karger publishers; 2020.
7. Mellors PW, Binder M, Ketterling RP, et al. Metaphase cytogenetics and plasma cell proliferation index for risk stratification in newly diagnosed multiple myeloma. Blood Advances. 2020;4(10):2236-44.
8. Mierla D, Malageanu M, Tulin R, et al. Prevalence of chromosomal abnormalities in infertile couples in Romania. Balkan J Med Genett. 2015;18(1):23-30.
9. Octavia Y, Hanafi MGS, Jazaldi F, et al. (2022). Patau syndrome: Genetic and epigenetic aspects. [online] Available from https://doi.org/10.2991/978-94-6463-062-6_32. [Last accessed November, 2024].
10. Pal AK, Ambulkar PS, Waghmare JE, et al. Chromosomal aberrations in couples with pregnancy loss: a retrospective study. J Hum Reprod Sci. 2018;11(3): 247-53.
11. Pozza C, Sesti F, Tenuta M, et al. Testicular dysfunction in 47, XXY boys: When it all begins. A semilongitudinal study. J Clin Endocrinol Metab. 2023;108(10): 2486-99.
12. Pylyp LY, Spynenko LO, Verhoglyad NV, et al. Chromosomal abnormalities in products of conception of first-trimester miscarriages detected by conventional cytogenetic analysis: a review of 1000 cases. J Assist Reprod Genet. 2018;35(2):265-71.
13. Shemilt L, Verbanis E, Schwenke J, et al. Karyotyping Human Chromosomes by Optical and X-Ray Ptychography Methods. Biophys J. 2015;108(3): 706-13.
14. Strome S, Bhalla N, Kamakaka R, et al. Clarifying Mendelian vs non-Mendelian inheritance. Genetics. 2024;227(3):iyae078.

CHAPTER 2

Basics of Pedigree Charting

Shruti Bajaj, Tasneem Shaikh, Niharika Jadeja

"A complete pedigree is often a work of great labour, and in its finished form is frequently a work of art"

—Karl Pearson, 1912

Q1. What is pedigree drawing?

Draft recommendations and evidence: In an era of increasing accessibility to sophisticated genetic tests, the century-old technique of pedigree elicitation still holds its relevance and value. A pedigree is a pictorial representation of a family's three-generational health history and genetic relationships, by utilizing standard symbols.

Q2. What are the standard symbols used in pedigree elicitation?

Draft recommendations and evidence: Standard nomenclature and symbols for human pedigree were first suggested in 1995. The important symbols relevant to obstetrics practice have been summarized in **Table 1**, in keeping with the revised recommendations. A detailed pedigree utilizes standard symbols to provide information about the affected individual (proband), the individual seeking consultation (consultand), age of onset of the disease, genetic results (if available) and consanguinity (if any).

Each generation of the pedigree should be depicted in the same horizontal plane. Each generation is defined by a Roman numeral (I, II, III), while each person in the particular generation is numbered with Arabic numeral (1,2,3) starting from the left **(Figs. 1 to 4)**. This enables easy to refer to multiple family members without necessarily knowing each individual's complete name.

Q3. What is the significance of pedigree charting?

Draft recommendations and evidence: Pedigrees offers valuable information about the family's medical history as well as relevant social relationships (divorced/single/death/adoption) which are essential for providing appropriate counseling recommendations. Careful depiction of a three-generational pedigree charting has been proven to detect 20% more individuals at risk of an inherited disease, as compared to a sole review of medical records.

The common modes of inheritances include Mendelian patterns **(Table 2)**, as well as non-Mendelian/nontraditional patterns (mitochondrial,

TABLE 1: Pedigree symbols.

Symbol depiction			
Significance	***Symbol***		
	Male	Female	Non-binary/ unknown
Person/ individual	 Name Age	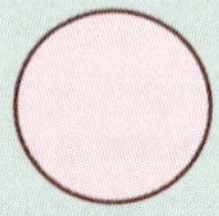 Name Age	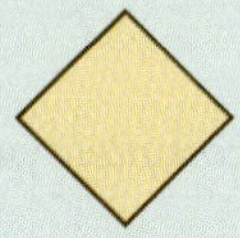 Name Age
Additional details about the person may be written in text below the symbol			
Significance	***Symbol***	***Significance***	***Symbol***
Multiple individuals (number known)	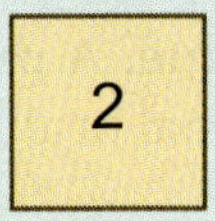	Multiple individuals (number not known)	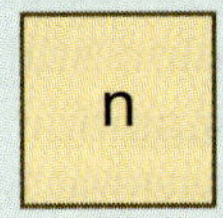
Proband	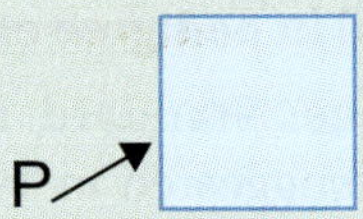	Consultand	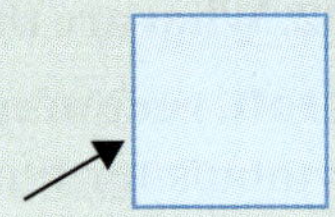
Proband is the affected individual that brings the family to medical attention. Consultand is the individual seeking genetic counseling. Sometimes, people mark consultand with a "C" near the arrow			
Disease status			
Affected individual	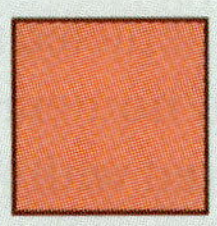 4 years	Affected with multiple conditions	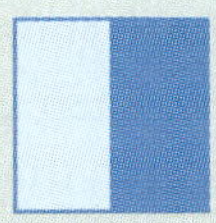 50 years
Patients can be affected with multiple conditions, as shown in the second figure. Remember to define shading in a key/legend			
Carrier 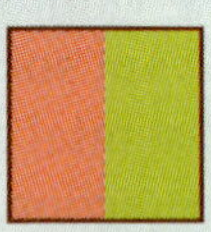 Autosomal recessive	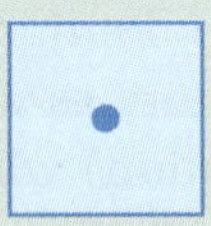 X-linked recessive	Deceased	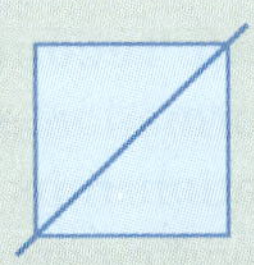 d. 75 years
For cases in which individuals are confirmed/obligate carriers of a genetic condition, we mark the pedigree with a dot		Age at death is recorded following "d"	

Contd...

Contd...

Pregnancy and outcomes			
Pregnancy	***Pregnancy loss***		***Stillbirth***
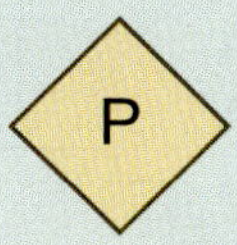 LMP: 2/4/24 GA: 16 weeks	Spontaneous abortion/ miscarriage	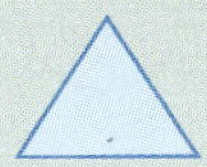 8 weeks	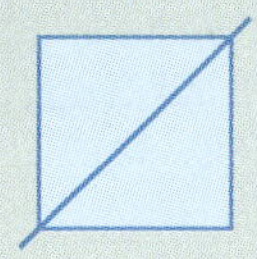 SB 34 weeks
	Ectopic pregnancy	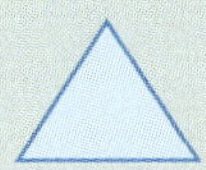 ECT	
	Medical termination of pregnancy	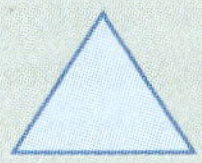 MTP	
Comments: Gestational age of the fetus is recorded below the symbol			
Multigestational pregnancies (twins, triplets, etc.)	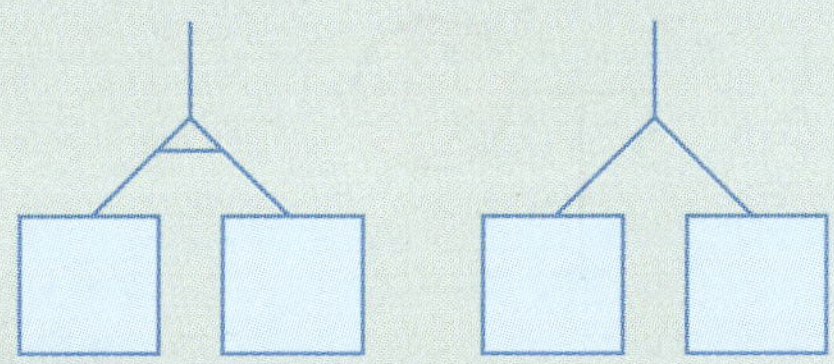		
Monozygotic twins should be represented by a connecting line unlike the dizygotic twins			

Relationship depictions	
Family relationship 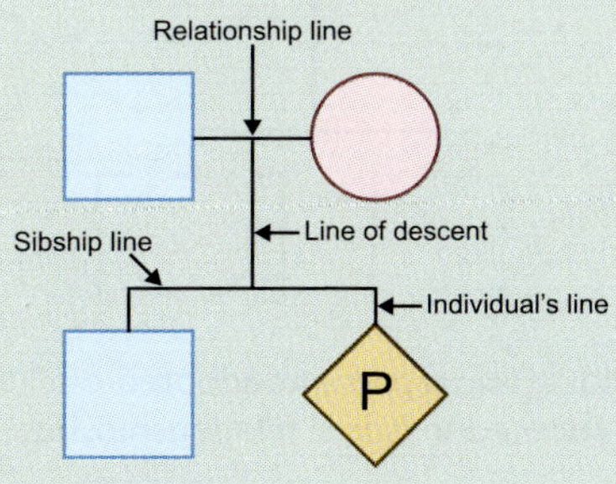	Divorce 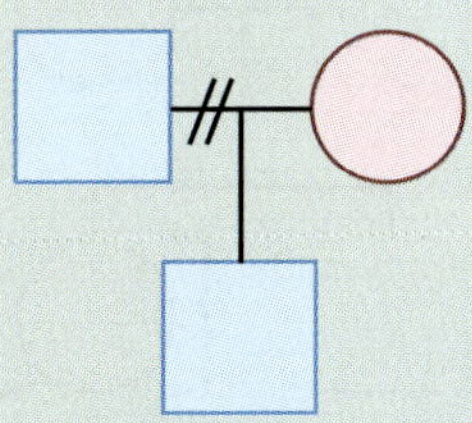
Siblings should be listed from left to right in birth order (oldest to youngest)	A break in a relationship line indicates the relationship no longer exists

Contd...

Contd...

Consanguinity

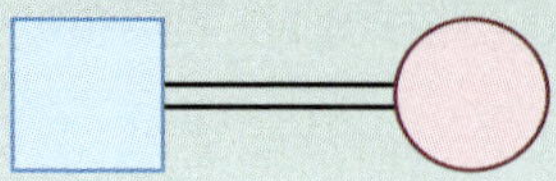

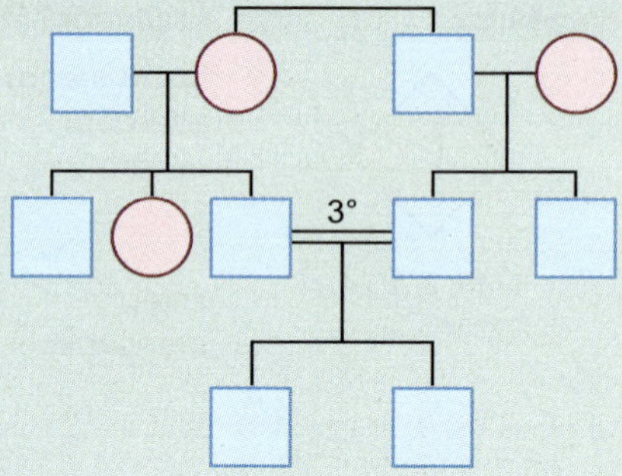

In general, consanguinity is represented as two lines connecting the partners. If aware of the nature of the relationship, it can be drawn out in the pedigree, with the degree of consanguinity mentioned above the relationship line

Children

No children by choice or reason unknown

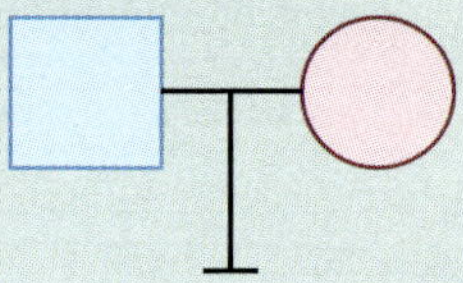

Infertility

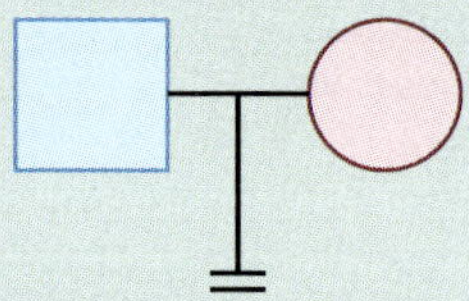

Indicate the reason if known below the two horizontal lines

Adoption

Adopted out

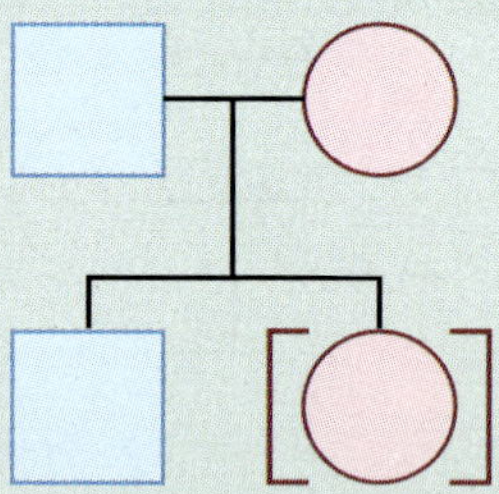

Adopted in

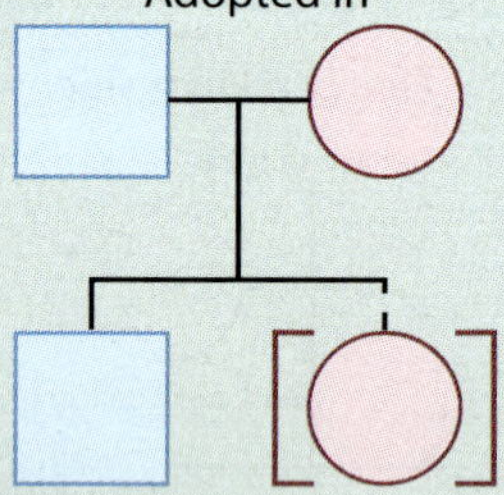

Brackets are used for all adoptions. Solid individual line represents adopted-out (genetic relationship). Dashed line represents adopted-in (social relationship, but not genetic)

Contd...

Contd...

Assisted reproductive technology/possible reproductive scenarios

Donor gametes

Egg donor

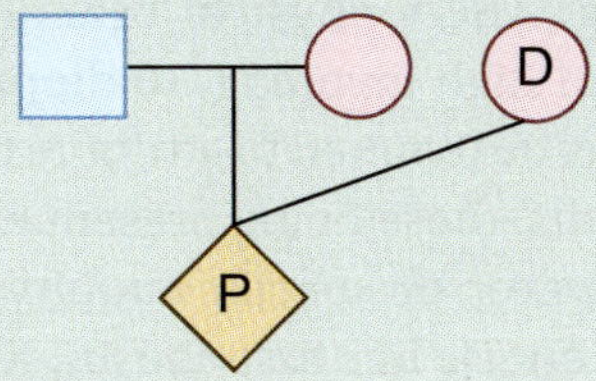

Sperm donor

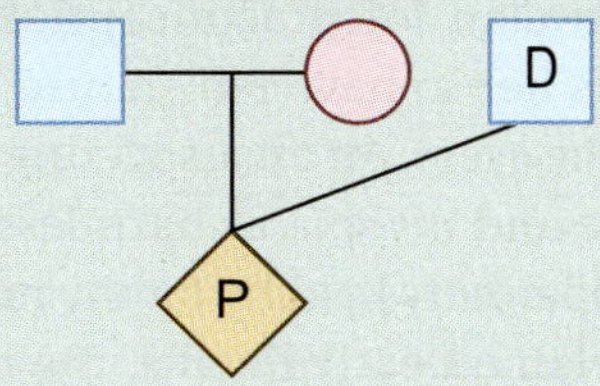

Notice how the pregnancy is connected to both the parents and the donor in the first example, because the female partner is carrying the pregnancy, even though she does not have a genetic relationship to the child. This is because there is still a biological relationship that can affect the fetus (e.g., teratogens, maternal disease). This is not the case in the second example, because the male partner does not have a biological relationship with the fetus

Both donor gametes

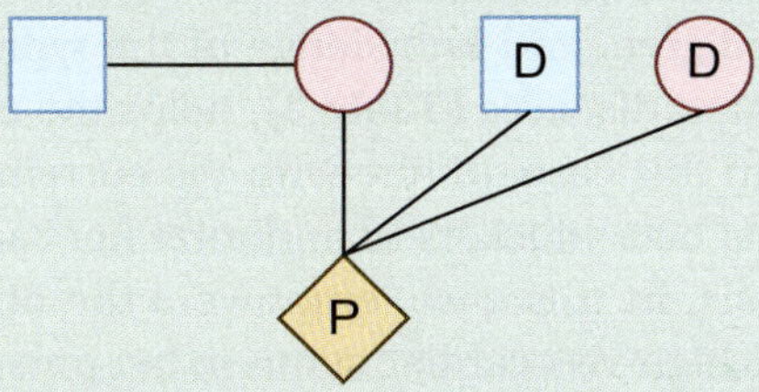

The pregnancy is conceived through an egg donor and sperm donor and carried by the female partner.

Surrogacy

Surrogacy with parental gametes

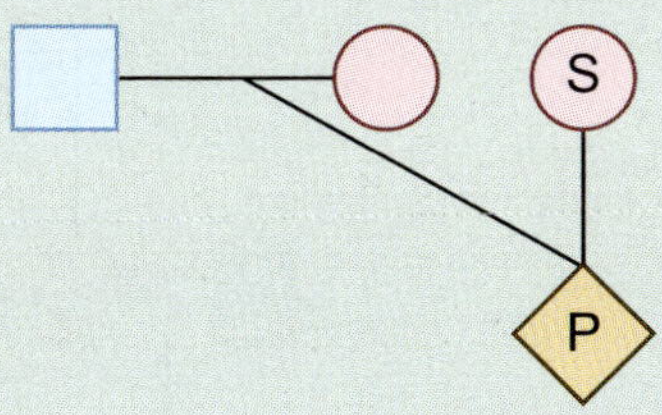

Surrogacy with ovum donor

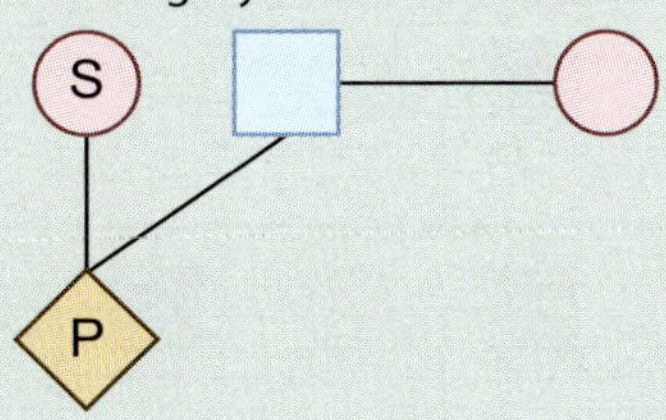

trinucleotide repeat expansion, polygenic inheritance, etc.). Let us try to understand the significance of pedigree charting through some simple case examples.

Case scenario 1 (Fig. 1): Mrs ABC (III-7), a 28-year-old lady, visits her obstetrician for preconception counseling. ABC's physical examination reveals her to have tall stature (184 cm) and high myopia (-10 diopters in both the eyes). An unsuspecting clinician may be tempted to attribute the tall stature and myopia as harmless 'familial traits', these being present even in the apparently healthy family members. However, on specific enquiry about unexplained early deaths, the consultand reports her first cousin, XY (III-2) succumbing from a cardiac arrest at the age of 32 years while trekking. His post-mortem autopsy mentioned aortic root dilatation. He too, like the consultand, had high myopia and tall stature. Subsequently, the clinician requested ABC's 2-dimensional echocardiogram, which reveals a dilated aortic root. Her genetic test reveals a pathogenic, heterozygous variant in *FBN1*, providing her with a diagnosis of Marfan syndrome. Intuitive history-taking based on the seemingly unrelated clinical clues, followed by a detailed elicitation of the pedigree, and knowledge of the typical clues suggestive of autosomal dominant diseases **(Table 2)**, helps the clinician arrive at an accurate diagnosis in this case. In line with the current recommendations, ABC is started on oral beta-blockers to minimize her cardiac complications. A complete diagnosis, in this case, empowers the obstetrician to better manage the patient's high-risk cardiac status in her prospective pregnancies. It also helps the family understand their reproductive options better, given the 50% risk of recurrence of the same disease in the future progeny. Notably, a detailed pedigree also helps the clinician enable cascade testing in the

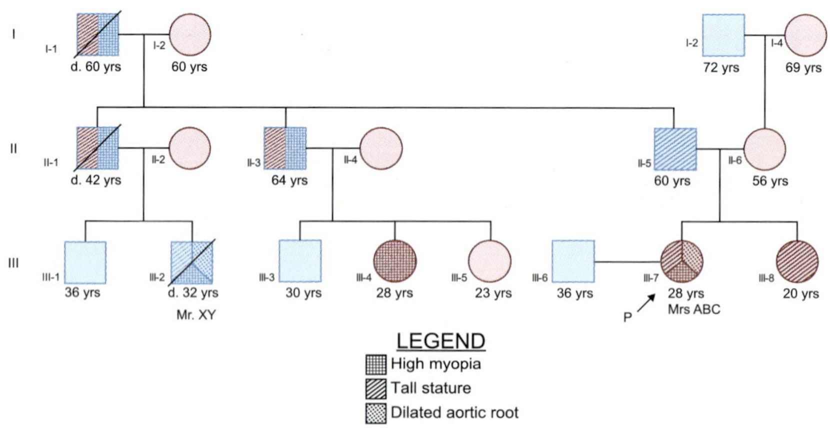

Fig. 1: Pedigree denoting autosomal dominant inheritance pattern (Marfan syndrome).

TABLE 2: Clues to recognize common Mendelian inheritance patterns.		
Autosomal dominant	***Autosomal recessive***	***X-linked recessive***
• The disease appears in every generation. Rarely generations may be skipped due to incomplete penetrance and variable expressivity • Males and females are equally affected • Male to male transmission occurs • 50% risk of recurrence in the future pregnancies	• The disease appears in the siblings, not in their parents • Males and females are equally likely to be affected • Usually consanguineous or endogamous union • 25% risk of recurrence in the future pregnancies	• The disease has a higher incidence in males • No father to son transmission • Females are obligate carriers and are usually unaffected • 50% of the males are affected • 50% of the females are carriers

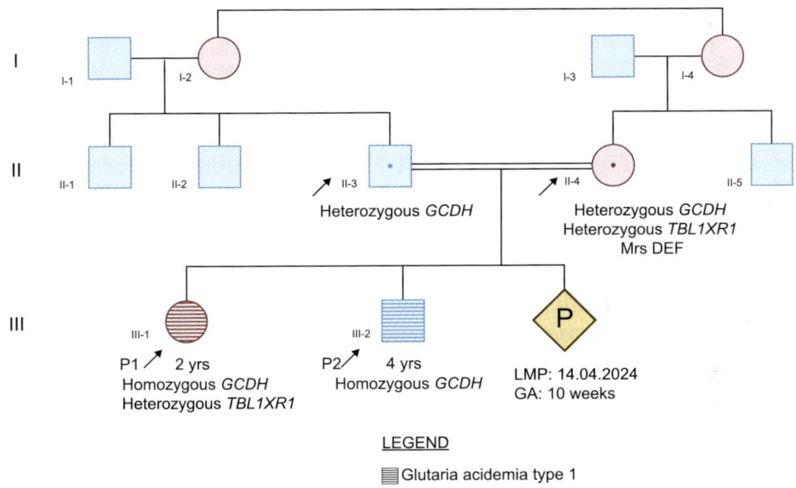

Fig. 2: Pedigree denoting autosomal recessive inheritance pattern (Glutaric acidemia).

patient's "as-yet unaffected but at-risk" family members (II-3, II-5, III-1, III-3, III-4, III-4, III-5, III-8), thus empowering them with early surveillance and reduced disease-related morbidity.

Case scenario 2 (Fig. 2): Mrs DEF (II-4) and her husband (II-3) are consanguineously married. They visit their obstetrician for prenatal genetic testing due to their previous two children (III-1, III-2) being affected with glutaric acidemia type I. During the pedigree elicitation, the husband claimed that the disease occurred in both the children due to their conception during a solar eclipse, considered to be associated with evil spirits in his culture. He detailed that '*no one in his seven generations was ever affected with a genetic disease*'. However, to the clinician, the pedigree typically suggests an autosomal recessive disease **(Table 2)**. The pedigree helps the clinician, in such scenarios to firstly, develop a patient rapport, while enabling him to understand the family myths in an empathetic manner. Interestingly, detailed review of the genetic reports reveals the elder child as well as the asymptomatic mother to harbor an additional variant of uncertain significance in *TBL1XR1* gene, known to be associated with autosomal dominant Pierpont syndrome. This finding, although uncertain, was potentially causing the mother to be blamed for the children's disease. Given that Pierpont syndrome is an autosomal dominant disease, with only *de novo* occurrences described in literature, the variant of uncertain significance in *TBL1XR1* segregating with the asymptomatic mother, seems irrelevant for disease causation as well as prenatal testing, in this scenario. Thus, the clinician offers prenatal testing for only glutaric acidemia, while noting a 25% risk of recurrence of the same disease in the current pregnancy. In this case, a simple and cost-effective pedigree along with logical clinical correlation helps the clinician navigate through complex patient belief systems, dissect through the variants of uncertain significance, and avoid unnecessary prenatal genetic testing of *TBL1XR1* variant, when not indicated.

Case scenario 3 (Fig. 3): Mrs PQR (III-2) meets her genetic professional due to a significant history of male members in her family being affected with an undiagnosed muscle-related disease that causes loss of ambulation and early mortality in the third decade of life. The clinical correlation and the pedigree **(Fig. 3)** make the geneticist suspect an X-linked disease **(Table 2)**, Duchenne muscular dystrophy (DMD), in this case. However, given the heterogeneous possibilities of genetic diseases which can present in a similar fashion, a definite diagnosis is necessary. The pedigree reveals the consultand's 14-year-old brother (III-1) to be available for genetic testing. *DMD* gene

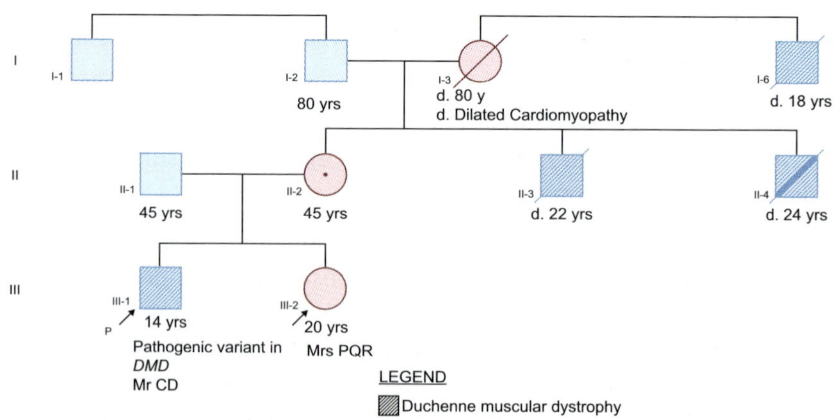

Fig. 3: Pedigree denoting X-linked recessive inheritance pattern (Duchenne muscular dystrophy).

targeted multiplex-ligation-probe-dependent-amplification (MLPA) confirms DMD in Mr CD (III-1). The same test enables the geneticist to rule out PQR's carrier status for DMD, thus, reassuring her. In this case, detailed pedigree elicitation helps to opt for the appropriate test in the appropriate person, and in the appropriate sequence. Since heterozygous female carriers of DMD are at risk of adulthood-onset dilated cardiomyopathy, a confirmed diagnosis, in this case, prompts the clinician to offer cardiac surveillance to other at-risk members (II-2).

Case scenario 4 (Fig. 4): Mr XYZ (III-1) meets a genetic professional to understand his risk of developing cancers, given his significant family history. Detailed history reveals that the father (II-2) was a chronic tobacco chewer since the age of 15-years. He was diagnosed of oral cancer at 50-years of age. The mother (II-3) succumbed at 46-years to bilateral ovarian cancer diagnosed in a premenopausal stage, barely a year before her death. Notably, her sister (II-4) has history of bilateral breast cancer, diagnosed at 48 years of age. To add, the consultand's maternal grandfather (I-3) had expired due to prostate cancer. The case highlights the importance of 'separating the unusual trees from the forest' and the role of pedigree charting in guiding the family, in such scenarios. While the father's cancer seems due to environmental factors and does not merit detailed genetic tests, the strong maternal history suggests a hereditary cancer predisposition syndrome (CPS). The sole living patient affected with a suspected CPS, II-4 in this case, is offered genetic testing. She is detected to harbor a heterozygous pathogenic variant in *BRCA1* gene. Predictive testing for the same in the consultand, after thorough pretest counseling, reveals him to be carrying the same variant in *BRCA1* gene. He is offered the appropriate onco-surveillance, based on these results.

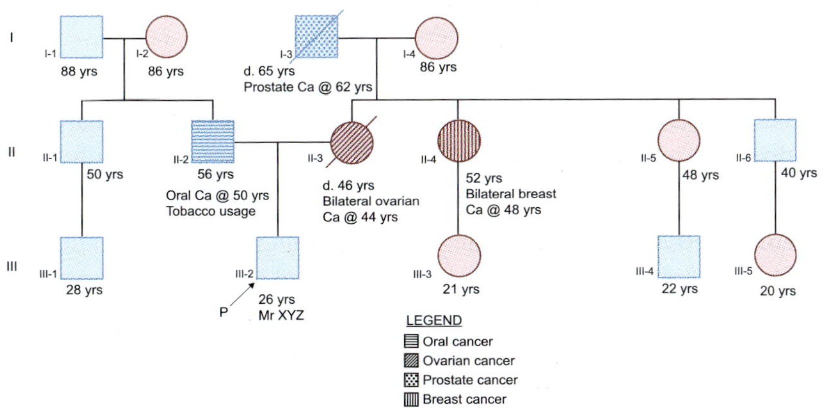

Fig. 4: Pedigree denoting non-genetic (tobacco) as well as genetic (*BRCA1*, autosomal dominant) inheritance patterns for cancer.

Based on the four case scenarios highlighted above, the significance of pedigree charting can be summarized as follows:

1. Pedigree as a diagnostic clue
2. *Assisting in the testing strategy:* Whom to test first? Which test? Are there more relatives at risk?
3. To establish pattern of inheritance and calculate the risks to the future generation as well as other family members
4. Distinguishing genetic from other risk factors
5. Tool to establish rapport with the patient family
6. *Assist in patient education:* A pedigree can help dispel myths, understand shared genetic as well as shared environmental risk factors, provide a visual clue about the 'at-risk' family members, help the patient in understanding the possible mode of inheritance
7. Interpretation of genetic reports, navigating through variants of uncertain significance.

Q4. What are the red flags to suspect a genetic disease?

We suggest a mnemonic '**Pedi-Green Flag'** (P-E-Di-G-R-E-E-N FL-A-G) to enable the clinician to suspect a genetic disease or a susceptibility to an inherited condition. Presence of one or more of the following clues should be a 'green flag' to alert the physician about referring the patient to a genetic professional.

P- Bilateral disease in **paired** organs (eyes, kidneys, hearing)

E- **Ethnicity**. Example: Beta thalassemia is seen more commonly in Kutchi, Bhanushali, and Sindhi communities from Western and Northwestern India than in other communities

DI- **Dysmorphlsms (facial dysmorphisms)**—especially if associated with neurodevelopmental concerns or other medical diagnosis

G- **Group of clinical features** that is evocative of a diagnosis. For example: Constellation of tall stature, arachnodactyly, myopia, aortic root dilatation in an individual should suggest a connective tissue disorder, commonly Marfan syndrome

R- **Reproductive concerns**—Infertility, multiple miscarriages, stillbirths, child deaths, premature ovarian insufficiency, and obstructive azoospermia. Example: Premature ovarian insufficiency can be due to premutation carrier state for Fragile X syndrome. Males with cystic fibrosis can present with azoospermia due to congenital bilateral absence of vas deferens.

E- **Earlier than usual onset of common diseases** (especially if multiple family members affected)

- Premenopausal breast cancer
- Prostate cancer <50–60 years
- Colon cancer <45–50 years
- Hearing loss <50–60 years
- Vision loss <55 years
- Heart disease <40–50 years
- Stroke <60 years

E- **Extreme/unusual manifestation of common presentation** (unusually severe fractures and multiple fractures after trivial trauma can be suggestive of metabolic or genetic bone disease, unusual obesity in <5 years age especially if associated with neurodevelopmental delays/visual concerns can be suggestive of monogenic diseases)

N- **Neurodevelopmental** concerns, progressive or unexplained neurological condition (seizures, tone abnormalities, ataxia, autism, learning difficulties, muscle weakness)

F-L- **FamiLy history**—Multiple closely related members with the same or related medical condition, particularly if rare. (Example: Family history of multiple members having early onset end-stage renal disease, and adulthood-onset obstructive cardiomyopathy along with acroparesthesias can suggest a diagnosis of Fabry's disease)

A- **Abnormal laboratory results:** Example: High value of HbA2 can indicate carrier state for beta thalassemia, low calcium values with hypoparathyroidism in a newborn with congenital heart disease can suggest 22q11.2 deletion syndrome

G- **Grouping of features:** Two or more medical conditions in the same person (Examples: Intellectual disability with cleft palate, two primary cancers), two or more major birth anomalies in the same individual/fetus, three or more minor anomalies in the same individual, three or more pregnancy losses.

BIBLIOGRAPHY

1. Benett RL. The Practical Guide to the Genetic Family History. 2nd edition. New Jersey: John Wiley & Sons; 2010.
2. Bennett RL, French KS, Resta RG, et al. Practice resource-focused revision: Standardized pedigree nomenclature update centered on sex and gender inclusivity: A practice resource of the National Society of Genetic Counselors. J Genet Couns. 2022;31(6):1238-48.
3. Bennett RL, Steinhaus KA, Uhrich SB, et al. Recommendations for standardized human pedigree nomenclature. Pedigree Standardization Task Force of the National Society of Genetic Counselors. Am J Hum Genet. 1995;56(3):745-52.
4. Committee Opinion No. 478: Family history as a risk assessment tool. Obstet Gynecol. 2011;117(3):747-50.

5. Dietz H. FBN1-related Marfan syndrome. In: Adam MP, Feldman J, Mirzaa GM, Pagon RA, Wallace SE, Bean LJ (Eds). GeneReviews® [Internet]. Seattle (WA): University of Washington, Seattle; 1993.
6. Frezzo TM, Rubinstein WS, Dunham D, Ormond KE. The genetic family history as a risk assessment tool in internal medicine. Genet Med Off J Am Coll Med Genet. 2003;5(2):84-91.
7. Solomon BD, Muenke M. When to suspect a genetic syndrome. Am Fam Physician. 2012;86(9):826-33.
8. Wright EMMB, Suri M, White SM, et al. Pierpont syndrome: a collaborative study. Am J Med Genet A. 2011;155A(9):2203-11.

3

CHAPTER

Preconception Carrier Screening for Genetic Disorders

Ratna Dua Puri

Q1. What is preconception carrier screening?

- Carriers are the individuals who are heterozygous for pathogenic or likely pathogenic variant in autosomal recessive or X-linked disorders
- Preconception carrier screening is the molecular testing performed on individuals and couples to find out the risk of having a child with an autosomal recessive or X-linked genetic disorder
- Carriers may be apparently healthy or may have some medical issues like premature ovarian failure in Fragile X syndrome.
- Carrier screening helps screened couples to consider their reproductive options, and to make informed decisions.

Q2. What is expanded carrier screening?

- Screening for a large number of genetic conditions simultaneously.
- Number of genetic conditions screened varies in different laboratories. These panels can screen for 5–10 conditions to several hundred conditions.
- These conditions should have:
    - Carrier frequency of 1 in 100 or more
    - Well-defined phenotype
    - Detrimental effect on quality of life
    - Cognitive or physical impairment that may need surgical or medical intervention
    - Screened conditions should be amenable to prenatal diagnosis

Q3. Who should be offered carrier screening in India?

Draft recommendation: All women planning a pregnancy and all pregnant women who are not screened preconceptionally should be offered carrier screening in India.

Summary of evidence: This is an acceptable strategy for carrier screening. Additionally ethnicity related or specific population related screening can also be offered if specific genetic disorders are reported in that ethnic group.

Q4. For what disorders should carrier screening be performed in India?

Draft recommendations:

- Universal carrier screening should be performed for ß thalassemia and other hemoglobinopathies and spinal muscular atrophy in India.

- As a second step, a detailed family history is taken to understand if the couples are at risk of being carriers based on the family history. In this situation, targeted carrier testing for the familial genetic variant is undertaken.
- Expanded carrier screening in India can be performed in specific situations like:
  - Consanguinity
  - Bad obstetric history with multiple pregnancies with ultrasound detected abnormalities where genetic testing for etiologic diagnosis has not be done.
  - Previous child with a suspected genetic disorder and where genetic testing was not done and the proband biological sample is not available.

Summary of evidence: There is abundant evidence for the carrier rate of ß thalassemia and other hemoglobinopathies in India and the pan ethnic carrier frequency of 3–4% has been well established in published literature. Studies for carrier frequency for spinal muscular atrophy in India are also now available and are reported between 1:30 to 1:44.

Information for the rest of the disorders is lacking with only very limited data available in literature. Additionally limitations for interpretation of identified variants as Indian mutation spectrum and normal population variants are not well represented in worldwide databases. As a result it is challenging to recommend universal expanded carrier screening for all autosomal recessive and X-linked disorders in India.

Q5. When should carrier screening be performed?

Draft recommendations: It is recommended that carrier screening should be performed before conception. However if the couple have not visited the doctor in the preconception period, it can be done in the first post conception visit, early in pregnancy. Concurrent testing of both partners can be done if there are time constraints.

Summary of evidence: There is a turnaround time for the results coupled with the need of preconception and post-conception counseling. If the fetus is found to be at risk for a genetic disorder for which prenatal testing is indicated, timelines to set up the specific mutation in the laboratory in preparation of the fetal sample must be factored in, along with the PCPNDT guidelines for pregnancy termination in India.

Q6. How should report of carrier screening be interpreted?

Draft recommendation and evidence: Only pathogenic and likely pathogenic variants should be reported in a carrier screening result.

The obstetrician/physician ordering the test should be able to understand the report generated by the laboratory. The laboratory must optimize the techniques used to generate the carrier screening report. The gene disease association and genetic variants and disease association must be established before prenatal testing is performed.

Q7. What is the role of pretest and post-test counseling for carrier screening?

Draft recommendations: Pretest and post-test counseling is mandatory before carrier screening test is ordered and after the results are received.

Summary of evidence: In pre-test counseling the couples are explained the reason for the test, the nature of the test, the outcomes of the test and the financial implications of the test. They are informed of the residual risk of a genetic disorder despite the carrier screening test.

Post-test genetic counseling includes details of the disease for which the couple are carriers and their offspring are at risk of inheriting, the option of prenatal testing including counseling if the fetus is reported affected.

Q8. When is referral to a clinical geneticist recommended?

Draft recommendations: A clinical geneticist referral is sought whenever the primary physician encounters situations of a positive family history or a high risk pregnancy based on the past history of the couple. Additionally referral is sought whenever the carrier screening report is ambiguous or variants of uncertain significance are reported.

Summary of evidence: A clear diagnosis is essential before invasive prenatal diagnosis is performed to avoid incorrect irreversible actions. Therefore referral must be taken in the event of unclear reports of carrier testing or positive family history or bad obstetric history to enable appropriate care for the couple.

Q9. Final statement regarding carrier screening.

Draft recommendations:

- Detailed family history must be taken for all couples.
- Carrier screening should be offered to all couples.
- Carrier screening is an optional test and it is not mandatory for the couple to consent to testing.
- It is the option of the couple for the number of diseases for which carrier testing is consented.
- Normal obstetric care must not be influenced by the decision of the couple for carrier screening.

BIBLIOGRAPHY

1. Balzotti M, Meng L, Muzzey D, et al. Clinical validity of expanded carrier screening: Evaluating the gene-disease relationship in more than 200 conditions. Hum Mutat. 2020;41(8):1365-71.
2. Committee Opinion No. 690: Carrier Screening in the Age of Genomic Medicine. Obstet Gynecol. 2017;129(3):e35-40.
3. Committee Opinion No. 691: Carrier Screening for Genetic Conditions. Obstet Gynecol. 2017;129(3):e41-55.
4. Gregg AR, Aarabi M, Klugman S, et al. Screening for autosomal recessive and X-linked conditions during pregnancy and preconception: a practice resource of the American College of Medical Genetics and Genomics (ACMG). Genet Med. 2021;23:1793-806.
5. Gregg AR, Aarabi M, Klugman S, et al. Screening for autosomal recessive and X-linked conditions during pregnancy and preconception: a practice resource of the American College of Medical Genetics and Genomics (ACMG). Genet Med. 2021;23:1793-806.
6. Kaur A, Kumari A, Kaur A, et al. Carrier frequency of spino-muscular atrophy in individuals of a reproductive age group from North India. J Family Med Prim Care. 2022;11(12):7870-4.
7. Nilay M, Moirangthem A, Saxena D, et al. Carrier frequency of SMN1-related spinal muscular atrophy in north Indian population: the need for population based screening program. Am J Med Genet A. 2021;185(1):274-7.
8. Sumedha D, Anita K. Prevalence of beta thalassemia carriers in India: a systematic review and meta-analysis. J Community Genet. 2023;14(6):527-41.
9. Verma IC, Kohli S, Shenbagam S, et al. Carrier screening of spinal muscular atrophy in north Indian population and its public health implications. Clin Genet. 2020;98:198-9.

CHAPTER 4

Ethical Considerations for Preconception Genetic Counseling in India

Bibhas Kar, Asmita Thakur

Q1. What is preconception genetic counseling, and what are its primary objectives in the Indian context, including compliance with the PCPNDT Act, 1994?

Draft recommendations:

- Genetic counseling is a communication process through which individuals who are either affected by, or may be at risk of developing a condition that may have a genetic basis, or are at risk of having children affected by such a condition, receive information and advice about its natural history and management, its transmission and the available reproductive options such as ART with preimplantation genetic diagnosis and adoption.
- Routine preconception genetic counseling should be offered to individuals or couples considering pregnancy particularly in regions with high rates of consanguineous marriages and inherited disorders.
- Counseling should include risk assessment based on past history, family history, including family history of diabetes, hypertension and history related to any genetic disorder running in family and its appropriate testing.
- Identifying individuals at risk of having children affected by genetic conditions or congenital anomalies allows counseling that aims to provide information on testing and its prevention in future pregnancy. This process takes place either at the preconception or early prenatal stage, although more options are available if risks are identified before the pregnancy.
- The PCPNDT Act, 1994, mandates strict protocols to prevent gender determination by any mean.

Summary of evidence: As per **ACOG 2019**, Women who presents for preconceptional counseling should be offered same genetic testing as indicated in pregnancy. As per **WHO 2012** Genetic conditions can be categorized as conditions that occur in specific areas or groups of people in which there is a family history, including consanguinity and disorders in one or both parents; and conditions identified in previous pregnancies should be addressed. The **PCPNDT Act, 1994** ensures that genetic counseling focuses on genetic disorders rather than sex determination to protect fetal rights. The **ICMR (2017) National Guidelines for ART Clinics** emphasize ethical practices in reproductive technologies, including genetic counseling, to prevent misuse and uphold high standards of care.

Research gaps: Despite recommendations for preconceptional genetic counseling there are less number of studies that are published to prove its utility and cost benefit analysis. Longitudinal studies are needed to evaluate the long-term outcomes of preconception genetic counseling on the health of offspring and the psychological well-being of parents.

Q2. What specific genetic tests are recommended in India for preconception counseling, and how do they identify risks for chromosomal disorders (trisomies, monosomies, and translocation) and single-gene disorders (autosomal dominant, autosomal recessive, and X-linked conditions)?

Draft recommendations:

- Routinely, no specific genetic testing is recommended in India in preconceptional period. However, screening for disease that are prevalent in the population and can easily be screened should be done. For example, hemoglobinopathies like sickle cell disease, beta thalassemia, etc., are endemic in India and the test recommended for carrier screening in prospective parents are MCV, high-performance liquid chromatography (HPLC) or Hb electrophoresis.
- In case of couple with history of recurrent spontaneous abortion, it is recommended to get chromosomal analysis of the couple to see for balanced translocation.
- On clinical examination and pedigree charting, if any genetic condition is suspected; it should be confirmed by a genetic test. Few example as detailed:

Clinical features	***Disease suspected***	***Test to be done***
Developmental delay, flat facies, open mouth, epicanthic fold	Down syndrome	Karyotype
Short stature, normal mental function, prominent forehead, trident hand	Achondroplasia	PCR-RFLP
Ambiguous genitalia	Congenital adrenal hyperplasia, 5α reductase deficiency	Karyotype, whole exome sequencing (WES)
Spinal deformity	Spondylocostal dysostosis	WES
Tall stature, history of lens dislocation, aortic regurgitation	Marfan syndrome	WES

Contd...

Contd...

Clinical features	*Disease suspected*	*Test to be done*
History of brother affected with mental retardation	Fragile X	*If brother can be tested:* Karyotype would commonly be normal. Fragile X syndrome diagnosis in the brother involves PCR and Southern blotting to assess CGG repeat expansions in the FMR1 gene
History of brother or maternal uncle is affected with muscle dystrophy (high CPK level)	Duchene muscular dystrophy	MLPA for DMD

- Genetic testing in one of the partner can be done for autosomal recessive carrier condition like Spinal muscular atrophy (SMA) and cystic fibrosis can be done by getting PCR and NGS on peripheral blood to detect specific mutations in the CFTR gene and SMN1 gene, respectively especially in consanguineous couple and/or couples with history of previous child death with respiratory failure.

Summary of evidence: Karyotyping is a well-established method for identifying numerical chromosomal abnormalities (Jackson et al., 2018). ACOG 2019 recommends universal screening for carrier status for Cystic fibrosis and spinal muscular atrophy by identifying mutation in CFTR gene and SMN1 gene.

Research gaps: Further research is needed to evaluate the effectiveness of current genetic screening programs in India, particularly in terms of their impact on reproductive decision-making and health outcomes. Research should focus on the integration of new genetic testing technologies and methodologies into existing healthcare frameworks to improve the accuracy and accessibility of genetic testing.

Q3. Which genetic disorders are most commonly screened for in the Indian population during preconception counseling, and what techniques and technologies are typically employed?

Draft recommendations:

- No genetic disorder is universally being screened in India.
- *Thalassemia screening:* Hemoglobin electrophoresis and high-performance liquid chromatography (HPLC) are recommended for detecting different types of hemoglobin and identifying carriers of

thalassemia. Regular screening should be implemented, especially in high-prevalence regions like Punjab and Gujarat.

- *Sickle cell anemia screening:* Hemoglobin electrophoresis should be used to identify hemoglobin S, while polymerase chain reaction (PCR) can confirm the presence of sickle cell traits. Screening should be prioritized in tribal areas and central India where the prevalence is high.
- *Cystic fibrosis screening:* PCR and genetic sequencing are advised for detecting mutations in the CFTR gene. Despite its lower prevalence, screening should be available for individuals with a family history or other risk factors.
- *Duchenne muscular dystrophy (DMD) screening:* PCR and Multiplex Ligation-Dependent Probe Amplification (MLPA) are recommended to identify mutations in the DMD gene. Early screening and diagnosis are crucial for effective management.
- *Fragile X syndrome screening:* PCR and Southern blotting should be used to detect CGG repeat expansions in the FMR1 gene. Screening should be considered for individuals with a family history of intellectual disabilities.
- *Down syndrome (Trisomy 21) screening:* Karyotyping and non-invasive prenatal screening (NIPS) are advised to detect chromosomal abnormalities. NIPS, which analyses fetal DNA, should be offered as a noninvasive alternative to traditional karyotyping.

Summary of evidence: The **ACOG 2019** recommends detailed family history of genetic disorder, birth defects, mental disorder, breast, ovarian, uterine and colon cancer should be taken. Also recommends universal testing for CFTR gene and SMN 1 gene mutation for cystic fibrosis and systemic muscular atrophy. Any women with h/o intellectual disability in family or ovarian insufficiency before 40 years should be offered testing for Fragile X chromosome. Hemoglobin electrophoresis and HPLC are effective for identifying carriers and differentiating types of hemoglobin in Thalassemia (Black et al., 2010).

Research gaps: Research on how emerging technologies, such as advanced sequencing methods, can be integrated into routine screening practices by reducing cost of test to enhance detection capabilities. Conduct studies to evaluate the long-term outcomes of genetic screening on individuals' health, reproductive decisions, and overall quality of life.

Q4. How is genetic counseling integrated with assisted reproductive technologies (ART) in India, and what measures ensure equitable access to genetic counseling and testing services for all populations?

Draft recommendations: Genetic counseling should be an integral part of ART procedures, including preconception and prenatal assessments, such as preimplantation genetic diagnosis (PGD). This integration helps ensure informed reproductive decisions by identifying genetic disorders in embryos before implantation.

Implement and enforce guidelines that require ART clinics to provide genetic counseling as a standard service, irrespective of socio-economic status. This regulation aims to reduce disparities in access to genetic services.

Summary of evidence: In India, genetic counseling is integrated with ART to provide comprehensive care by offering preconception and prenatal genetic assessments. Preimplantation genetic testing (PGT) is a key component, screening embryos for genetic disorders before implantation. The Indian Council of Medical Research (ICMR) guidelines emphasize that genetic counseling must be part of ART clinic protocols, ensuring informed decision-making for couples undergoing ART procedures. **The ICMR** guidelines mandate that ART clinics must offer genetic counseling to all couples, aiming to reduce the disease burden.

The National Program for Prevention and Control of Cancer, Diabetes, Cardiovascular Diseases, and Stroke (NPCDCS) supports efforts to increase awareness and access to genetic services, especially in underserved regions. Efforts to enhance genetic service accessibility include expanding outreach programs and training genetic counselors to reach rural and remote areas, thereby improving the inclusivity and availability of these services across diverse populations.

Research gaps: There is a need for further research to evaluate the effectiveness of integrating genetic counseling with ART in improving reproductive outcomes and decision-making. The current practice of pre implantation genetic testing for both aneuploidy and single gene disorder needs objectification and publication with follow up of such fetuses after delivery.

Q5. What considerations are necessary for ethnic-specific genetic screening in India, and how do family history and consanguinity impact genetic risk assessment?

Draft recommendations:

- Ethnic background associated with an increased prevalence of a heritable disorder (e.g., beta thalassemia is a prevalent hemoglobinopathy in Sindhis (carrier status of 17%), sickle cell disease in tribal area of Maharashtra, Odisha and Madhya Pradesh, HbE disease in north-eastern state etc.
- Develop targeted genetic screening programs that address the prevalence of specific genetic disorders within different ethnic and regional populations. For example, include thalassemia screening in regions like Punjab and Gujarat, and sickle cell anemia screening in tribal areas.

- Consanguinity increases the risk of autosomal recessive disorder. Implement more intensive screening protocols for autosomal recessive disorders in communities with high rates of consanguineous marriages. This should include increased awareness and testing for conditions prevalent in these populations.
- Utilize detailed family history as a critical tool in genetic risk assessment. Tailor genetic testing and counseling based on familial patterns of genetic disorders, even if these conditions are not prevalent in the general population.

Summary of evidence: Ethnic-specific genetic screening in India is crucial due to the country's diverse genetic landscape. Certain genetic disorders are more common in specific ethnic groups due to historical, geographical, and cultural factors. For instance, thalassemia is prevalent in Punjab and Gujarat, while sickle cell anemia is more common in tribal regions. Tailoring screening programs to these regional and ethnic variations ensures effective identification of at-risk individuals.

Consanguinity, prevalent in some Indian communities, increases the likelihood of autosomal recessive disorders because of the higher probability of inheriting the same genetic mutations from both parents. This practice necessitates more rigorous screening for recessive conditions.

Research gaps: Further research is needed to evaluate the effectiveness of ethnic-specific genetic screening programs in improving the identification and management of genetic disorders. Studies should explore the impact of tailored screening panels on early diagnosis and prevention within various ethnic groups. More research is required to understand the implications of consanguinity on the prevalence and management of autosomal recessive disorders.

Q6. Why is it crucial to address the psychosocial impact of genetic testing results on prospective parents, and how is informed consent ensured while safeguarding confidentiality and privacy?

Draft recommendations:

- Implement a thorough informed consent process that clearly explains the purpose, risks, benefits, and limitations of genetic testing.
- The apprehension of being carrier of a genetic defect may lead to marital dispute, depression, stress, anxiety and emotional distress related to genetic risk information.
- Provide comprehensive psychosocial support and counseling for prospective parents undergoing genetic testing.
- Ensure that prospective parents understand the potential emotional impact of test results and provide them with adequate time to make an informed decision.

- Adhere to strict protocols for handling genetic data, including anonymizing information, limiting access to authorized personnel, and using secure storage and transmission methods.
- Clearly communicate to individuals how their genetic information will be used, stored, and shared, and obtain their consent for these practices.

Summary of evidence: Informed consent is fundamental in genetic testing, ensuring that individuals fully understand the implications of the tests. Effective informed consent helps individuals make voluntary and well-informed decisions. Confidentiality and privacy are critical in protecting sensitive genetic information and maintaining trust between patients and healthcare providers.

Q7. What steps are taken to comply with national and international ethical and legal guidelines in genetic counseling, and how are cultural, religious, and social contexts incorporated into the counseling process in India?

Draft recommendations:

- Ensure that informed consent is obtained from patients by providing comprehensive information about the purpose, nature, risks, benefits, and potential outcomes of genetic testing.
- Confidentiality must be maintained rigorously to protect patient privacy, in alignment with the ICMR's National Guidelines for Accreditation, Supervision & Regulation of ART Clinics (2017).
- Adapt genetic counseling practices to accommodate India's diverse cultural and religious beliefs. This includes understanding and respecting community-specific practices and attitudes toward genetic disorders and reproductive choices, especially in communities with high rates of consanguinity.
- Tailor the counseling process to reflect the values and beliefs of individuals and communities. This approach helps build trust and improves the effectiveness of genetic counseling by addressing specific needs and preferences of patients.
- Implement cascade screening programs to test family members of individuals with known genetic disorders.
- Suspected X-linked condition, the female partner consent needs to be asked before counseling the couple together. The documentation needs to be written and given to patient with written consent.

Evidence: To align with both national and international guidelines in genetic counseling, it is crucial to follow ethical and legal standards, including obtaining informed consent and maintaining confidentiality. The ACOG Committee Opinions (2005, 2009) and the ICMR National Guidelines (2017) emphasize these principles.

Cultural, religious, and social contexts are integral to effective genetic counseling in India's diverse population. Practices must be adapted to respect community-specific beliefs, particularly in areas with high consanguinity. Public health initiatives, like NPCDCS, aim to enhance awareness and access to genetic services, addressing disparities and incorporating cultural considerations.

Q8. How are ethical dilemmas related to reproductive choices, such as selective abortion or preimplantation genetic testing (PGT), addressed, and how are reproductive options discussed with prospective parents?

Draft recommendations:

- *Selective Abortion:* Adhere to the Medical Termination of Pregnancy (MTP) Act (1971, amended 2021), which permits abortion under specific conditions, including severe fetal abnormalities detected before 24 weeks of gestation. Comprehensive counseling should be provided to discuss the moral, ethical, and psychological impacts of selective abortion, ensuring that parents make informed decisions without coercion.
- *Pre-implantation Genetic Testing (PGT):* Address ethical concerns associated with PGT, such as embryo biopsy safety, the risk of misdiagnosis due to mosaicism, and the moral status of embryos. Trophectoderm biopsy is preferred due to lower risks, and confirmatory tests like amniocentesis are often recommended to ensure accuracy (Harton et al., 2017).

Evidence:

- *Guidelines for PGT:* ACOG (2020) emphasizes informed consent, patient autonomy, and non-directive counseling in PGT. ASRM (2023) focuses on managing PGT for monogenic conditions, ensuring patient understanding. ESHRE (2020) provides good practice recommendations, including lab standards and ethics. HFEA (UK) regulates PGT for ethical and legal compliance, while the Indian Society for Assisted Reproduction (2021) promotes ethical use in IVF with comprehensive counseling. Ethical views on embryos are varied, necessitating non-directive counseling to respect diverse perspectives and inform prospective parents about PGT and selective abortion.
- *Guidelines and Regulatory Compliance for PGT:* ACOG Opinions (2006, 2009) and ICMR Guidelines (2017) emphasize the critical importance of informed consent and confidentiality in genetic testing, including PGT. Adherence to ACMG standards ensures accuracy in genetic testing and counseling, while the PCPNDT Act (1994) regulates prenatal diagnostics to prevent misuse for sex selection, ensuring ethical practices.
- Guidelines from ACOG, ASRM, ESHRE, and the Indian Society for Assisted Reproduction provide frameworks for these issues, emphasizing informed consent, patient autonomy, and ethical practice.

Q9. What role does Non-Invasive Prenatal Screening (NIPS) play in preconception genetic counseling in India, and how does it compare with traditional invasive diagnostic methods in terms of accuracy, safety, and accessibility?

Draft recommendations:

- There is no role of NIPS in pre conceptional genetic counseling; however, NIPS can be performed for prenatal genetic screening.
- NIPS or cell free DNA is the most sensitive and specific screening test for the common fetal aneuploidy, it is safe and accessible but it can be false-positive or false-negative. Furthermore, cell-free DNA testing is not equivalent to diagnostic testing.
- Incorporate NIPS as a standard option in prenatal care protocols to provide early and non-invasive risk assessment for chromosomal abnormalities. Ensure comprehensive counseling is provided to prospective parents regarding the benefits, limitations, and implications of NIPS results.
- Diagnostic testing which is to be done by invasive procedures such as chorionic villous sampling, amniocentesis or cordocentesis has diagnostic accuracy of 100%. But as it is invasive procedure, small risk of abortion, bleeding or leaking is there.

Summary of evidence: The NIPS offers a safer and more accurate alternative to traditional invasive diagnostic methods for assessing the risk of chromosomal abnormalities. NIPS analyses cell-free fetal DNA in maternal blood, providing high sensitivity and specificity, with detection rates for conditions like Down syndrome, Trisomy 18, and Trisomy 13 exceeding 99%. Unlike invasive procedures such as amniocentesis and chorionic villus sampling (CVS), which carry a risk of miscarriage (0.25% to 1.0%), NIPS does not involve any physical risk to the fetus or mother. In India, NIPS was introduced in 2012 and is preferred in private healthcare settings despite its higher cost and initial limited availability. The PCPNDT Act regulates its use to prevent sex-selective abortion and restricts fetal sex disclosure to cases of detected genetic abnormalities. While NIPS enhances early prenatal care and decision-making, its accessibility remains a challenge, particularly in rural areas. Efforts are underway to improve NIPS availability through public health initiatives and integration into broader healthcare practices.

The ACOG recommends prenatal genetic **screening** (serum screening with or without nuchal translucency, ultrasound or cell-free DNA screening) and **diagnostic** testing (chorionic villus sampling or amniocentesis) options should be discussed and offered to all pregnant patients regardless of maternal age or risk of chromosomal abnormality.

Patients with a negative screening test result should be made aware that this substantially decreases their risk of the targeted aneuploidy but does not ensure that the fetus is unaffected. The potential for a fetus to be affected by genetic disorders that are not evaluated by the screening or diagnostic test should also be reviewed.

Research gaps: Further research is needed to explore strategies for reducing the cost of NIPS and increasing its availability in underserved regions. Its sensitivity in both low risk and high risk population needs more deliberations.

Q10. How does preconception genetic counseling address the prevention of genetic diseases through lifestyle modifications and early interventions, and what public health initiatives support these efforts in India?

Draft recommendations:

- Integrate lifestyle recommendations into preconception genetic counseling, including advice on diet, exercise, and avoidance of harmful substances.
- Provide advice for individuals at risk, such as folic acid supplementation for neural tube defects or dietary adjustments for metabolic disorders.
- Implement comprehensive genetic screening programs, including cascade and carrier testing, to identify at-risk individuals and couples.
- Couple with suspected genetic disorder or history of previous fetus or child with malformation, recurrent perinatal mortalities, previous fetus with suspected genetic syndrome or previous child with GDD, these couple preferably tested in inter conception period so that in next pregnancy early prenatal testing can be done.

Summary of evidence: Preconception genetic counseling is instrumental in preventing genetic diseases by incorporating lifestyle modifications and early interventions. Genetic risk assessments guide personalized recommendations, such as lifestyle changes for managing conditions linked to genetic predispositions and preventive measures like folic acid supplementation for reducing the risk of neural tube defects. Early interventions, including genetic screening and carrier testing, enable informed reproductive choices and the use of ART and PGD to prevent genetic disorders. Public health initiatives in India, such as the National Programme for Prevention and Control of Cancer, Diabetes, Cardiovascular Diseases & Stroke (NPCDCS), the National Health Mission (NHM), and the Integrated Child Development Services (ICDS), support these efforts by integrating preconception care into broader health programs and enhancing access to preventive services.

Research gaps: Basic training to treating obstetrician about genetic testing and counseling so that patient can be referred to fetal medicine specialist or genetic specialist for counseling and testing.

Increase access to genetic counseling and screening services across diverse populations, especially in rural and underserved areas.

BIBLIOGRAPHY

1. ACOG Committee Opinion No. 762 Summary: Prepregnancy counseling. Obstet Gynecol. 2019;133(1):228-30.
2. Black ML, Sinha S, Agarwal S, et al. A descriptive profile of β-thalassaemia mutations in India, Pakistan and Sri Lanka. J Community Genet. 2010;1(3): 149-57.
3. Colah RB, Mukherjee MB, Martin S, et al. Sickle cell disease in tribal populations in India. Indian J Med Res. 2015;141(5):509-15.
4. Committee on Genetics, American College of Obstetricians and Gynecologists. ACOG Committee Opinion. Number 325, December 2005. Update on carrier screening for cystic fibrosis. Obstet Gynecol. 2005;106(5):1465-8.
5. Committee on Gynecologic Practice. ACOG Committee Opinion No. 727: Cascade Testing: Testing Women for Known Hereditary Genetic Mutations Associated With Cancer. Obstet Gynecol. 2018;131(1):e31-4.
6. Coonen E, Rubio C, Christopikou D, et al. ESHRE PGT Consortium good practice recommendations for the detection of structural and numerical chromosomal aberrations. Hum Reprod Open. 2020;2020(3):hoaa017.
7. Guha S, Reddi HV, Aarabi M; ACMG Laboratory Quality Assurance Committee. Laboratory testing for preconception/prenatal carrier screening: a technical standard of the American College of Medical Genetics and Genomics (ACMG). Genet Med. 2024;26(7):101137.
8. Harton GL, Cinnioglu C, Fiorentino F. Current experience concerning mosaic embryos diagnosed during preimplantation genetic screening. Fertil Steril. 2017;107(5):1113-9.
9. Indian Council of Medical Research (ICMR). National Ethical Guidelines for Biomedical and Health Research Involving Human Participants. New Delhi: Indian Council of Medical Research; 2017.
10. Indian Council of Medical Research (ICMR). National Guidelines for Accreditation, Supervision, and Regulation of ART Clinics in India. New Delhi: Indian Council of Medical Research; 2017.
11. Ioannides AS. Preconception and prenatal genetic counselling. Best Pract Res Clin Obstet Gynaecol. 2017;42:2-10.
12. Jackson M, Marks L, May GH, et al. The genetic basis of disease. Essays Biochem 2018;62(5):643-723.
13. Jayashankar SS, Nasaruddin ML, Hassan MF, et al. Non-Invasive Prenatal Testing (NIPT): Reliability, Challenges, and Future Directions. Diagnostics (Basel). 2023;13(15):2570.
14. Kumar SH, Athimoolam K, Suraj M, et al. Comprehensive genetic analysis of 961 unrelated duchenne muscular dystrophy patients: focus on diagnosis, prevention and therapeutic possibilities. PLoS One. 2020;15(6): e0232654.
15. Malhotra J, Malhotra K, Majumdar G, et al. Indian Society for Assisted Reproduction Consensus Guidelines on Preimplantation Genetic Testing in In vitro Fertilization Clinics. J Hum Reprod Sci. 2021;14(Suppl 1):S31-47.
16. Olney RS, Moore CA, Khoury MJ, et al. Chorionic villus sampling and amniocentesis: recommendations for prenatal counseling. MMWR Recomm Rep. 1995;44(RR-9):1-12.

17. Practice Committee and Genetic Counseling Professional Group of the American Society for Reproductive Medicine, American Society for Reproductive Medicine, Washington, D.C. Indications and management of preimplantation genetic testing for monogenic conditions: a committee opinion. Fertil Steril. 2023;120(1):61-71.
18. Preimplantation Genetic Testing: ACOG Committee Opinion, Number 799. Obstet Gynecol. 2020;135(3):e133-7.
19. Singh S, Thakur S. Preconception and prenatal screening for common genetic disorders in India. AOGD Bulletin. 2019;18(1):8-10.

5

CHAPTER

Prenatal Screening and Invasive Testing

Vandana Bansal, Rupal Parekh Tulle, Palak Sharma

Q1. Is prenatal genetic screening a selective approach for high-risk pregnancy or a universal approach to all pregnancies?

Draft recommendations: All pregnant women should be offered aneuploidy screening irrespective of maternal age and history.

Summary of evidence: Every woman has a risk that her fetus has a chromosomal defect. Chromosomal abnormalities are present in about 0.9% of newborns and include numerical or structural chromosomal abnormalities. Overall risk of Down's syndrome in general population is about 1 in 800 pregnancies. Rates of abnormalities are higher among stillbirths and miscarriages. Chromosomal anomalies are responsible for more than half of the miscarriages, and a large majority of these (90%) are numerical, particularly autosomal trisomies (involving chromosomes 13, 16, 18, 21, 22), polyploidy and monosomy X.

Because of association of advancing maternal age with meiotic chromosomal nondisjunction in oocyte predisposing to aneuploidy, prenatal diagnosis has traditionally been offered to women at 35 years of age or older for many years. As maternal age advances, risk of having child with Down's syndrome increases from about 1 in 1000 at 30 years of age, to almost 1 in 400 at 35 years of age, and 1 in 100 at 40 years of age. In spite of these statistics Down's syndrome is discovered at birth in more younger age patients than older pregnant women because of larger population of pregnant women belonging to younger age group. Screening for only the older subgroup of pregnant patient will detect only 30% of Down's syndrome. Therefore, maternal age alone is no longer used as a definite indication for screening or invasive testing. Aneuploidy screening in pregnancy is offered to all irrespective of maternal age.

It is very important to explain the optional nature of all prenatal testing and to emphasize this fact that a low-risk screening test result does not guarantee a healthy child and a high risk screening test result does not mean the fetus has the disorder. Distinction should be made clear between a diagnostic and a screening test. A screening test identifies an increased likelihood of a fetal abnormality in an apparently normal pregnancy whereas a diagnostic test confirms or refutes the existence of an actual anomaly in a fetus believed to be at increased risk.

Q2. What are the screening tests available for aneuploidy in the prenatal period and which one is the best screening modality (biochemical or sonographic or combination of both)?

Draft recommendations:

- Combined first trimester screening (cFTS test) should be offered as a standard of care to all antenatal women at 11-13+6 weeks of gestation regardless of maternal age.
- Where expertise for assessment of all soft markers in the first trimester is not available, first trimester screen (FTS) which includes Nuchal Translucency along with dual marker should be used.
- Biochemical Markers alone (Dual Marker or Triple marker) are not recommended as a screen test due to its low sensitivity.
- If the first trimester screen is missed, second trimester screening should be offered at 15–21 weeks of gestation which includes biochemical markers (quadruple marker) and genetic sonogram.
- First trimester screen should not be followed by a second trimester screen independent of each other. If necessary, both need to be integrated for a better sensitivity.
- NIPS is an optional screening test for high-risk patients including maternal age 35 years or older at delivery, previous pregnancy affected with trisomy, positive screening results for aneuploidy, including first trimester, sequential, integrated, or quadruple screen.

Summary of evidence: Biochemical and sonographic tests differ as per weeks of gestation.

1. *First trimester biochemical screening for aneuploidy: Double marker test* is a biochemical screen which includes maternal serum free beta human chorionic gonadotropin (β-hCG) and pregnancy associated plasma protein A (PAPP-A), both produced by placenta. It is carried out between 11 and 13^{+6} weeks gestation, equivalent to a crown rump length of 45–84 mm **(Table 1)**. Dual marker alone should not be used for screening as the detection rate is low.
2. *First trimester screening test (FTS)* is a terminology used for a combination of maternal age, dual marker screen along with nuchal translucency at a

TABLE 1: Values of individual biochemistry in Dual marker test.

Dual marker parameters	*PAPP-A*	*Free β-hCG*
Trisomy 21	Decreased ≤0.5 MoM	Increased ≥2.0 MoM
Trisomy 18	Decreased	Decreased
Trisomy 13	Decreased	Decreased
Sex chromosome abnormality	Decreased	Normal

crown rump length of 45–84 mm. This gives a risk assessment for trisomy 21, 13, and 18. The detection rate of this First trimester screen test is >90% for a 5% false-positive rate. Regardless of maternal age first trimester screening test is offered as a standard of care to all at 11–13^{+6} weeks.

3. *Combined First trimester screening (cFTS):* Effectiveness of the first trimester screening is improved further if along with nuchal translucency, other first trimester markers such as fetal nasal bone, assessment of blood flow across tricuspid valve, fetal heart rate and ductus venosus flow are included. Addition of these first trimester markers increase detection rate for Trisomy 21 to more than 95% for a false positive rate of 2.5% and 95% with false positive rate of 0.1% for Trisomy 13 and 18.

   In a prospective validation study, the first-trimester combined test detected 90%, 97%, and 92% of trisomies 21, 18, and 13, respectively, as well as 95% of cases of monosomy X and triploidies and >50% of other chromosomal abnormalities, at a FPR of 4%. In a women with previous history of fetus or infant with Down's syndrome, risk of recurrence in subsequent pregnancy increases by 0.75% over and above the risk calculated by maternal age (a priori risk) or risk calculate from combined first trimester screen.

4. *Second trimester biochemical screening for aneuploidy:* Quadruple test includes a combination of four biochemical serum markers, i.e., free beta hCG, MSAFP, unconjugated estriol (uE3), and inhibin A. This test is used to screen for trisomy 21, 18, and neural tube defects between 15 and 21 weeks. Detection rate of quad screen is between 81 and 85.8% for false positive rates of 7–8.3% as compared to triple test with low detection rate of only 69% which is now obsolete. In cases where first trimester screen could not be done, quadruple test should be offered owing to its better detection rates and lower false positive rates. In pregnancies affected with trisomy 21, elevated levels of hCG, inhibin A and reduced levels of MSAFP, uE3 are observed.

   Maternal serum alpha-fetoprotein (MSAFP) levels in the quadruple test are elevated in women with fetus having open neural tube defects. Other fetal conditions that have been associated with elevated MSAFP levels are; abdominal wall defects, oligohydramnios, renal or chromosomal abnormalities. Placental dysfunction leading to obstetric complications later in gestation such as preterm birth, preeclampsia, and fetal growth restriction, may also cause an increase in MSAFP levels. First trimester multifetal pregnancy reduction or spontaneous single fetal demise in multiple pregnancy has been found to cause persistent elevation in MSAFP levels. Several factors other than gestational age affect MSAFP levels include maternal weight, race, insulin dependent diabetes mellitus, and the number of fetuses.

With better ultrasound technology and better training and technique, sensitivity of ultrasound for the detection of NTD and other structural anomalies associated with raised MSAFP levels is as high as 94 to100%. Hence measurement of amniotic fluid AFP and acetylcholine esterase is optional with a 97% detection rate for NTDs with a FPR of 0.5%.

The timing of various screening tests and the detection rates have been summarized in **Tables 2 and 3**.

5. *Combined first and second trimester screening:* With the aim of improving detection rate, first trimester combined screening is followed by second trimester biochemical screening and results of both trimester screening tests are combined and risk is calculated. Two approaches have been defined integrated test and sequential screening.

   In *integrated test*, first trimester combined screening is followed by second trimester quadruple marker screening and combined results

TABLE 2: Various screening tests and the timing of the tests available.

Screening test	***Gestational age***	***Parameters tested***
Combined first trimester screen/first trimester screen	11–13.6 weeks (45–84 mm)	Nuchal translucency with dual marker (free β-hCG and pregnancy-associated plasma protein-A) with or without nasal bone, flow in ductus venosus, tricuspid regurgitation
Quadruple screen	15–22 weeks	• Free β-hCG • Alpha fetoprotein (AFP) • Unconjugated estriol (uE3) • Dimeric inhibin A
Integrated screening	• First trimester screen • Quadruple screen	Reports of first trimester screen withheld, given as single risk estimate after quadruple screen
Sequential screening	• First trimester screen • Quadruple screen	• First trimester screen reports disclosed • Risk estimate given as high risk or low/intermediate risk • All high risk are offered diagnostic test and low/intermediate risk are offered NIPS or quadruple screen
Contingent screening	• First trimester screen • Quadruple screen	• First trimester screen reports disclosed. • Risk estimate given as high, intermediate, or low risk. High risk are offered invasive testing, low risk are followed up and intermediate risk are offered further testing like NIPS or quadruple screen
Noninvasive prenatal screening (NIPS)	Any time after 9 weeks	Evaluation of cell-free fetal DNA in maternal circulation. Risk estimate given as high risk or low risk

TABLE 3: The detection rate of all screening methods.

Method of screening	*Detection rate (%)*	*False positive rate (%)*
Maternal age (MA)	30	5
First trimester		
MA + fetal NT	75–80	5
MA + dual marker test	60–70	5
MA + NT + dual marker test (FTS)	85–95	5
FTS + nasal bone/tricuspid flow/ductus venosus flow (cFTS)	93–96	2.5
Second trimester		
MA + triple test	60–65	5
MA + quadruple test	81–85	5
MA + NT + PAPP-A (11–13 weeks) + quadruple test	90–94	5
Genetic sonogram alone	59	5
Combined first trimester screening with second trimester biochemical testing		
Integrated screening	90–94	5
Step-wise sequential screening	90–94	5
Contingent screening	90–94	5
Noninvasive prenatal screening	99.8%	<1

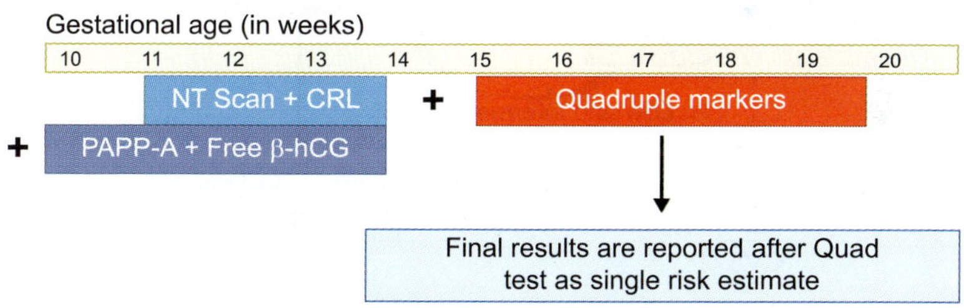

Fig. 1: Integrated test (timing and technique).

are given after completion of process in second trimester and pregnant women who fall into high-risk group, undergo invasive diagnostic testing by amniocentesis. This screening strategy combines results of first and second trimester marker screens and final risk is assigned after both tests are done. In population with limited access to CVS, serum integrated testing can be more acceptable with highest detection rate and lowest false positive rates. However, there is a longer wait time (3–4 weeks) between initiation and completion of screening, which may cause increased anxiety in the patients **(Fig. 1)**.

Sequential screening test are of two types: stepwise and contingent. Here the report is disclosed to the patient after the first trimester screen results.

In *step-wise sequential screening*, all patients undergo first trimester combined testing and on the basis of screening results, they are assigned three risk categories; low, intermediate and high risk. High risk cases receive genetic counseling and are offered invasive testing by chorionic villous sampling (CVS) whereas low and intermediate risk patients undergo quadruple screening in second trimester and if the combined risk after first and second trimester testing is high, the patients are offered amniocentesis **(Fig. 2)**.

The second approach is *contingent screening* which is similar to stepwise sequential testing, but second trimester biochemical screening is performed only in intermediate risk group after first trimester combined screening followed by final combined risk assessment in the second trimester. With contingent screening, pregnancy is classified as low, intermediate, or high risk based on first trimester screening results. Women at high risk are offered CVS. Women at intermediate risk are offered continued screening in the second trimester and women at low risk have no further testing **(Fig. 3)**. Theoretically, contingent screening would maintain a higher detection rate while reducing the number of patients undergoing second trimester screening tests.

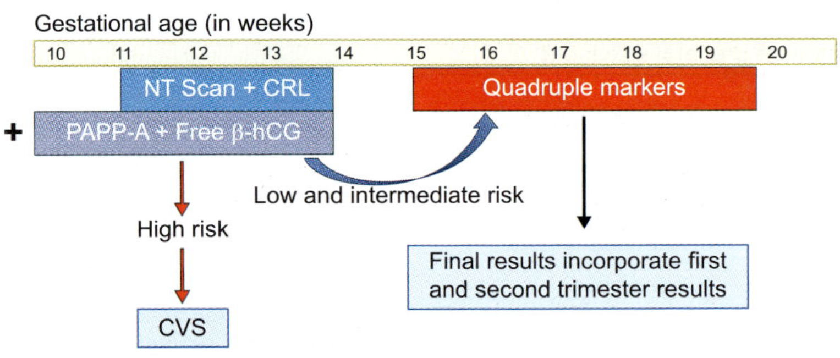

Fig. 2: Stepwise sequential test (timing and technique).

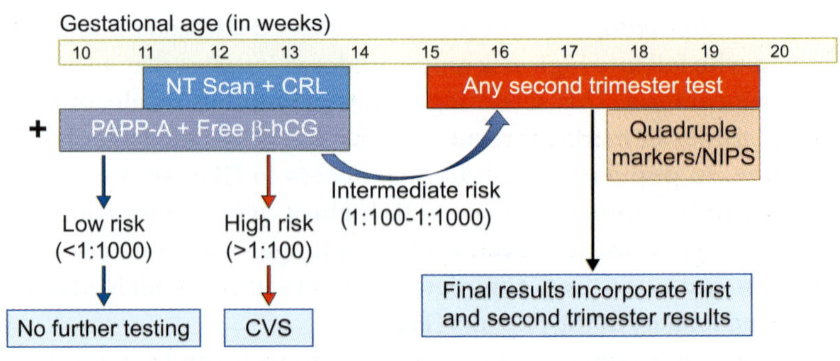

Fig. 3: Contingent test (timing and technique).

6. *Noninvasive prenatal screening (NIPS):* Noninvasive prenatal screening (NIPS) is an advanced screening test with high sensitivity and specificity for knowing the risk for fetal chromosomal aneuploidy using cell free DNA from maternal serum. Maternal plasma has approximately 5% to 20% of cell free DNA that comes predominantly from placental apoptosis which is fetal in origin.

   Testing can be performed starting as early as 9 weeks and until delivery. The sensitivity and specificity of this test varies with the platform used. Overall sensitivity and specificity reported for trisomy 21 is 99.3% and 99.8% respectively for a false positive rate of <1%. This makes this test an attractive alternative to traditional serum screening for aneuploidy. Recently with the advancement in the NGS technique few other applications including other aneuploidies and some microdeletions/duplications can also be detected but at a low accuracy.

   Main limiting factor to its widespread use as a screening method is its cost as well as chance of inability of getting a report if the fetal fraction is low. At present, SMFM (Society for Maternal Fetal Medicine) has recommended NIPS as the most appropriate screening test for high-risk patients including maternal age 35 years or older at delivery, previous pregnancy affected with trisomy, positive screening results for aneuploidy, including first trimester, sequential, integrated, or quadruple screen. In presence of fetal structural anomaly, decision for fetal karyotyping and or microarray testing should not be deferred by a normal NIPS result. NIPS is not a diagnostic test and confirmatory invasive testing is required in the presence of any abnormal screening results.

   Flowchart for various types of screening tests and the diagnostic tests have been shown in **Flowchart 1**.

Flowchart 1: Types of screening and diagnostic tests for aneuploidy.

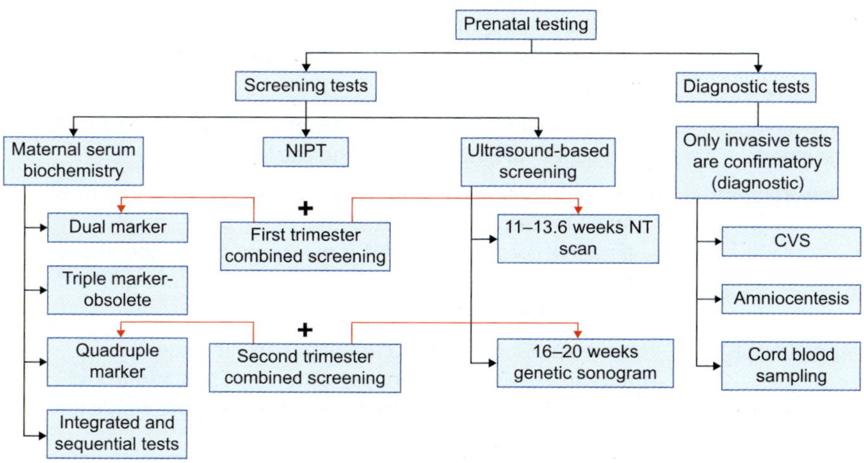

Q3. What are the criteria for nuchal translucency measurement? How does it affect first trimester screening?

Draft recommendations:

- Nuchal translucency (NT) is an objective evaluation on ultrasound of subcutaneous fluid behind the fetal head, neck and torso in the first trimester of pregnancy between 11^{+0} and 13^{+6} weeks of gestation, equivalent to a crown rump length of 45–84 mm.
- Stringent criteria must be followed to measure nuchal translucency (The Fetal Medicine Foundation criteria). This will ensure a universal and standardized manner of assessment and will help achieve uniformity of results for aneuploidy screening **(Table 4)**.

Summary of evidence: NT measurement is the single most effective screening test for fetal aneuploidy. Maternal age combined with nuchal

TABLE 4: FMF criteria for nuchal translucency.

USG machine	***High resolution with a video-loop and caliper that provides measurement to one decimal point***
Gestational age	11^{+0} weeks to 13^{+6} weeks
Crown rump length	45–84 mm
Magnification	Fetal head and torso occupy 75% of image
Position	• Midsagittal view of fetus with fetus facing toward transducer • Neutral position, neither hyper extended nor hyper flexed
Anatomical landmarks	• Tip of the nose, hard palate is trapezoid in shape • Absence of frontal process of maxilla (zygoma) • Rounded hypoechoic structure within center of intracranial cavity representing thalamus • Amniotic membrane to be differentiated from nuchal skin by waiting for spontaneous fetal movement or by tapping the mothers' abdomen or coughing to make the fetus jump
Caliper placement	Horizontal cross-hatch of the caliper should be flushed with the inner aspect of the line bordering the NT
Measurement	• Perform three measurements and largest measurement is taken for risk assessment • If nuchal cord is present NT is measured below and above the cord and average of the two is taken. Reduce gain before measurement to reduce fuzzy edge of the line
Appearance	It is the amount of fluid accumulation (NT thickness) and not its appearance (presence or absence of septation/fluid accumulation confined to neck or enveloping the whole fetus) that determine risk

translucency alone provides detection rates of 75% for fetus affected by trisomy 21 for a false positive rate of 5%.

Increased nuchal thickness is not a numerical cut off value, rather it is the measurement relative to the specific crown rump length. The measured NT must first be converted to gestational age specific multiples of the median (MoM). The MoM values are integrated in dual marker analysis for the first trimester screening. Therefore the NT values directly affect the dual marker risk calculation; also implying that accurate measurement is of crucial importance for prenatal screening (and false measurement can lead to underestimate or overestimate risk of aneuploidy).

Using a combination of maternal age and NT, similar detection rates are achieved for trisomy 13 and 18, 90% for monosomy X and 60% for triploidy. The combined first trimester screen (cFTS) method which includes nuchal translucency, maternal dual marker and other first trimester markers (nasal bone/ductus venosus waveform/tricuspid regurgitation) reduces the invasive testing rate drastically to <3% and increases the detection rate for Down's syndrome and other chromosomal defects to >95%.

Q4. What else is detectable on NT scan? What are additional markers on NT scan? Are there stringent criteria for these markers?

Draft recommendations:

- Effectiveness of the first trimester screening is improved further if along with nuchal translucency, other first trimester markers such as fetal nasal bone, assessment of blood flow across tricuspid valve, fetal heart rate, and ductus venosus flow are included.
- First trimester uterine artery Doppler alone or in combination with PAPP-A and PLGF should be done in the 11-13+6 weeks NT scan to screen for risk of preeclampsia.
- 70–80% of major structural anomalies can be detected during the NT scan
- Pregnancy complications including preeclampsia, fetal growth restriction, chorionicity in multiple gestations, and preterm delivery can be predicted.
- Fetuses with NT above 99th centile must be evaluated for malformations, congenital heart defects, genetic syndromes and should undergo invasive testing for aneuploidy as well as chromosomal microarray.

Summary of evidence: Even if conventional karyotyping is normal, increased NT is predictive of adverse pregnancy outcome, because it is associated with other genetic aberrations like micro deletion/duplication syndromes, structural fetal malformations, congenital heart defects, intrauterine death and miscarriages. The risk is proportional to the nuchal translucency thickness and especially when NT measurement is 3.5 mm or more. These chromosomally normal fetuses with an enlarged NT require meticulous evaluation by a detailed ultrasound examination and echocardiography.

Meta-analysis on increased NT in 2020 indicated that in fetus with raised NT, 1:7.4 fetuses a chromosomal aberration was diagnosed. Of these aberrant cases, 69% involved trisomy 21, 18, and 13 and would potentially be detected by all NIPT approaches. The residual risk is for microdeletion or duplication which can be detected by microarray test.

Additional first trimester ultrasound markers for aneuploidy

1. *Absent nasal bone:* In about 60–70% of fetuses with trisomy 21, 50% of trisomy 18, 45% of trisomy 13 and in 2% of euploid fetuses, nasal bone is not visualized/ossified at 11–13 weeks. Nasal bone is affected by ethnicity and is higher in Black and Asian population and least in Caucasians.

   Nasal bone is evaluated in the same standard plane as for nuchal translucency during the same $11–13^{+6}$ weeks. It is seen as two echogenic lines roughly parallel to each other (equal sign) and should be as echogenic as skin.
2. *Reversed a-wave in ductus venosus:* Reversed a-wave during atrial contraction is observed in 3% of euploid fetus and in about 66% of fetuses with trisomy 21, 55% of trisomy 13 and 18 and 75% of fetuses with monosomy X **(Table 5)**.
3. *Tricuspid regurgitation:* Tricuspid valve regurgitation is seen in 55% of trisomy 21, 30–38% in trisomy 13, 18 and monosomy X. Abnormality of tricuspid regurgitation may also be seen in fetuses with cardiac defects. Tricuspid regurgitation may also be seen in 1% of normal fetuses **(Table 6)**.

Structural anomalies in the first trimester can be classified into:

a. Always detectable—anencephaly, body stalk anomaly, alobar holoprosencephaly
b. Potentially detectable—congenital diaphragmatic hernia, cardiac defects, neural tube defects

TABLE 5: How to measure a-wave in ductus venosus.

Position	Right parasagittal view of fetal upper abdomen
Magnification	Abdomen and thorax occupying majority of the image
Identifying DV	On color Doppler aliasing seen in vessel connecting hepatic portion of umbilical vein with inferior vena cava is the ductus venosus
Sample gate	Small sample gate (0.5–1 mm) in order to avoid contamination with hepatic veins and artery
Angle of insonation	<30°

TABLE 6: How to assess tricuspid regurgitation.	
Position	Transverse 4 chamber heart
Magnification	Chest occupies 75% of the image
Doppler sample	• Doppler gate placed across tricuspid valve • Large sample size used (2–3 mm)
Angle of insonation	<30%
Normal waveform	Biphasic waveform with first wave due to forward flow during diastole and second larger wave due to atrial systole
Tricuspid regurgitation	During ventricular systole any backward flow across tricuspid valve is considered regurgitation if the peak velocity of the regurgitant jet is >60 cm/s and should remain for at least 30% of ventricular systole

c. Not detectable—microcephaly, hydrocephalus, echogenic lung lesions, agenesis of corpus callosum

Q5. What is a genetic sonogram? Which are the soft markers for aneuploidy in second trimester? How to integrate soft markers in risk assessment?

Draft recommendations:

- Genetic sonogram is a standard of care for all antenatal cases.
- The soft markers that significantly increase the likelihood of trisomy 21 are thickened nuchal fold, borderline ventriculomegaly, absent or hypoplastic nasal bone, echogenic bowel, aberrant right subclavian artery.
- If any soft marker is detected then the likelihood ratio of aneuploidy for that soft marker should be multiplied by the a-priori risk (Maternal age based or prior screen risk based) for the pregnancy and couple should be counseled for need of further genetic testing depending on the posterior risk.

Evidence:

Second trimester genetic sonogram: A detailed ultrasonography for fetal anatomic survey is commonly used as an aneuploidy screening method in the second trimester which is usually best performed between 18 and 22 weeks of gestation. Approximately one third of fetuses affected with trisomy 21 have a major or minor structural variation identifiable on USG. Major abnormalities associated with Down syndrome are congenital heart defects, ventriculomegaly and duodenal atresia. Chromosomal defects are also associated with certain second trimester sonographic features (also known as soft markers), including biometric parameters (e.g., short length of femur and humerus, pyelectasis, increased nuchal fold, ventriculomegaly, hypoplastic or absent nasal bone, early fetal growth

TABLE 7: Soft marker likelihood ratios.

Marker	*LR+*	*LR-*	*Isolated marker LR*
Absent or hypoplastic nasal bone	23.27	0.46	6.58
Aberrant right subclavian artery	21.48	0.71	3.94
Increased nuchal fold thickness	23.3	0.8	3.79
Ventriculomegaly	27.52	0.94	3.81
Echogenic bowel	11.44	0.9	1.65
Mild pyelectasis	7.63	0.92	1.08
Intracardiac echogenic focus	5.83	0.8	0.95
Short femur/humerus	3.72	0.8	0.61

restriction) and morphologic signs (e.g., choroid plexus cysts, echogenic bowel, and echogenic intracardiac focus).These "soft markers" are physical characteristics which are not themselves abnormalities or defects but occur more commonly in fetuses affected with Down syndrome. Each soft marker is associated with a risk (likelihood ratio) for genetic abnormality. The likelihood ratio is calculated by dividing the percentage of chromosomally abnormal fetuses by the percentage of chromosomally normal fetuses with the same measurement. The likelihood ratio for every marker present in fetus can be used to modify the a priori risk or serum screening risk which forms the basis for ultrasound screening for Down syndrome. The pregnancy-specific risk of trisomy 21 is calculated by multiplying the *a priori* risk (maternal age and gestation dependent) by the likelihood ratio of each sonographic or biochemical measurement for the same pregnancy **(Table 7)**.

The detection of any of the above markers during a routine sonogram warrants careful anatomical survey aimed at identifying additional markers because the finding of multiple markers indicates high risk for chromosomal anomaly. The soft markers that significantly increase the likelihood of trisomy 21 are thickened nuchal fold, borderline ventriculomegaly, absent or hypoplastic nasal bone, echogenic bowel, aberrant right subclavian artery. Genetic sonogram alone has a detection rate of 69% with a 5% false-positive rate and enhances the sensitivity of all other screening methods. Relying only on USG to identify Down syndrome is not recommended.

Q6. What cut off should be used for screening to label the screen as screen positive? Should intermediate risk be acted upon?

Draft recommendations:

- A risk greater than 1:250 is screen positive and less than 1:1000 is low risk. A risk between 1:250 and 1:1000 is intermediate risk.

- Intermediate risk on a FTS or a quadruple test with no abnormality on first trimester scan or an anomaly scan may be given an option of NIPS to further stratify their risk.

Summary of evidence: Not many evidence based recommendations are available for management of intermediate risk group. A study in Asian population suggests that NIPT can be is used as a next step after intermediate risk is detected on FTS to further stratify their risk. This is based on the rationale to reduce the number of invasive procedures. They suggested that older women (i.e., aged ≥ 35 years) should be informed that the false-positive rate of FTS is higher for them than for younger women. Women who have intermediate risk are more likely to undergo invasive diagnostic testing. Among women with intermediate risk (1:250–1,000) the number of invasive tests per case of trisomy 21 was 13.5 (2 cases detected for 27 procedures performed). Detection rate for trisomy 21 in women aged ≥35 years (85.7%) was slightly lower than that of women aged <35 years (87.5%). This study also suggests that NIPT has role of benefit in older women (age ≥35 years) since the false positive rate of FTS is higher in older women (age ≥35 ears) than for younger women.

Q7. What are the screening methods for twin gestation and their detection rates? Is the interpretation different depending on chorionicity? Can we do prenatal screening in Triplet and higher order gestation, reduced fetus/single demise?

Draft recommendations:

- Nuchal translucency along with additional soft markers combined with first trimester biochemical screening is the most useful screening tool for multiple pregnancies as it can evaluate each fetus individually due to different NT and CRL.
- Screening for twin gestation depends on the chorionicity
- In MCDA twins (monozygotic) risk for aneuploidy is pregnancy-specific and is calculated by an average of NT measurement of both fetuses along with dual marker.
- In DCDA, risk assigned is fetus-specific and two separate risks are given depending on individual nuchal translucency.
- Maternal serum biochemistry for aneuploidy alone does not perform well in multiple pregnancy (both in the first or second trimester)
- NT assessment along with additional soft markers is the most useful and the only screening option in high-order pregnancies or pregnancies with reduced fetus/single demise.
- Screening for structural anomaly is equally important along with genetic screening in twin pregnancy.

Summary of evidence:

Prenatal screening in multiple gestation: In dizygotic twins, the fetal risk of Down's syndrome is independent of each other whereas in monozygotic twins, both are most commonly either affected or unaffected. As per the ISUOG guidelines for routine screening in twins, Combined first trimester screening can be used for trisomy 21. Alternative is using only combination of maternal age plus NT (without maternal serum markers).

National Collaborating Center for Women and Children suggested that the detection rate for Down syndrome may be lower in twin compared with singleton pregnancy with first-trimester screening. A recent meta-analysis reported similar performance [89% for singletons, 86% for dichorionic twins and 87% for monochorionic twins, at a false-positive rate (FPR) of 5%]. The pooled sensitivity of the test was 89.3%, with a pooled specificity of 94.6% for the detection of Trisomy 21. The performance of comprehensive first-trimester genetic screening in twin gestations for trisomy 13 and trisomy 18 has not been well described in the literature, presumably due to the low number of affected fetuses.

As regards to quadruple marker screening for trisomy 21 in twin gestation the studies show variable results. One meta-analysis reported the trisomy 21 detection rate to be as low as 47%. The variable results may be due to that abnormal analytes related to an affected twin may be masked by the presence of normal screening analytes in the unaffected cotwin.

Screening methods in case of vanishing twin/fetal demise: A vanishing twin can affect maternal serum values up to 4–6 weeks after fetal demise. Hence maternal serum based screening methods can be used after this time window or an alternative method is using only NT + maternal age for risk prediction. In case of a vanished twin, if there is still a measurable fetal pole, NT alone, in combination with maternal age, should be used for risk estimation.

NIPT is less accurate in case of vanishing twin. NIPT can be used >8 weeks after fetal cardiac activity is absent.

Screening for structural anomaly: Monozygotic twins are two to three times more likely to be affected by fetal anomaly, so fetal anatomy scan, including fetal echocardiography, is essential in every case. If only one fetus in a twin gestation is affected then it is said to be a discordant anomaly.

Q8. What is the next step after high risk screen report (NIPS or invasive)?

Draft recommendations:

- Invasive prenatal diagnosis continues to be the gold standard for pregnancies at increased risk for chromosomal anomaly or other genetic disorders.

- However if diagnostic testing facility is not available or patient does not desire invasive procedure then NIPT can be offered (ACOG guidelines for NIPT). However individual case-based assessment is a must.
- NIPT may be offered when risk is solely on serum markers provided that no other significant history or no structural defects seen on ultrasound. At the same time patient to be counseled about the limitations of NIPT.

Summary of evidence: When high risk is detected on screening test, then gold standard test for confirmation is invasive testing which includes amniocentesis, chorionic villus sampling and fetal blood sampling.

Q9. What are the indications and prerequisites for performing amniocentesis/CVS/cordocentesis?

Draft recommendation and evidence: Currently valid indications for invasive prenatal testing include increased risk for fetal chromosomal abnormality, increased risk for hereditary genetic or metabolic disease and increased risk for some perinatal infections.

Indications for invasive fetal testing:

- *Increased risk of fetal aneuploidy:*
  - Abnormal prenatal screening test results from first trimester combined screening/NIPS/second trimester triple or quadruple test
  - Abnormal ultrasound findings like fetal structural anomaly or multiple soft markers associated with aneuploidy
  - Previous fetus or child affected by aneuploidy
  - Parental aneuploidy or mosaicism for aneuploidy or parental carrier of chromosomal balanced translocation or inversion.

    *Advanced maternal age >35 years alone should not be considered an indication. Conception by assisted reproductive techniques in itself is again not considered a valid indication for invasive prenatal diagnosis.
- *Increased risk for a known genetic or biochemical disease of the fetus:*
  - History of family hereditary disease with a known mutation or biochemical change
  - Male fetus and carrier status of pregnant woman for a disease with X-chromosomal inheritance
  - Carrier status of both parents for an autosomal recessive disorder
- *Maternal transmissible infectious disease:* History of maternal primary infection or seroconversion involving toxoplasma, cytomegalovirus or rubella

Prerequisites to be followed while performing genetic tests include:

1. The test should be selected depending on the indication of the test, gestational age, and the information sorted

2. Recognized center and person performing prenatal invasive procedures
3. Ultrasound diagnosis and blood group and typing
4. Appropriate pretest counseling should be given to the couple regarding the turnaround time, limitations, sensitivity, specificity, and positive and negative predictive values of the test.
5. Post-test counseling regarding the result of the test and information regarding any further testing, including familial testing, support and follow-up in the present pregnancy and future pregnancies, if any should be provided to the couple.
6. Specimen should be provided in adequate quantity with optimum quality in an appropriate container and medium to allow for proper testing, depending on the test requested
7. Storage of genetic material may be recommended for further tests, should the need arise
8. Maternal blood sample should be provided to rule out maternal cell contamination

Q10. Which are the invasive methods available, their technique and their complication rate? What are the genetic tests that can be sent from the prenatal sample?

Draft recommendation and evidence:

Amniocentesis:

- Amniocentesis refers to transabdominal aspiration of amniotic fluid (around 15–30 mL) from the uterine cavity using 20–22 G spinal needle under continuous ultrasound guidance avoiding placental and cord insertion site and involves obtaining fetal skin cells from the amniotic fluid for culture for fetal karyotyping.
- It is recommended to perform amniocentesis at or beyond 15 + 0 weeks of gestation (ISUOG and CDC guidelines) as higher rate of total fetal losses, fetal talipes and post-procedure amniotic fluid leakage is reported in cases of early amniocentesis done before 14 weeks.
- Needle entry through the placental cord insertion site must be avoided and, if technically feasible, avoidance of the placenta is preferable, especially in Rhesus-negative women.
- Complications include risk of fetal loss varying from 0.1 to 1% (miscarriage rates for amniocentesis range from 0.25 to 0.5%) postprocedure membrane rupture in 1–2%, chorioamnionitis <1%, needle injury to the fetus and maternal sepsis in very rare circumstances. Less experience in invasive procedures, multiple attempts, blood-stained amniotic fluid and the presence of fetal abnormalities may increase the risk for fetal loss.

- In case of amniocentesis performed in later gestation in the third trimester, the risk of preterm labor is 3–4% (RCOG guidelines).

Chorionic villous sampling:
- CVS is the withdrawal of trophoblastic cells from the placenta performed between 11 and 14 weeks of gestation by transabdominal or transcervical route according to operator's preference or placental location using 18–20 G needle under continuous ultrasound guidance.
- It is recommended not to perform CVS before 10 completed weeks of gestation, due to higher risk of fetal loss and complications like limb reduction defects/oromandibular hypoplasia.
- Complications include fetal loss (0.2–2%), vaginal bleeding (10%, 30% after transcervical), amniotic fluid leakage (<0.5%) and chorioamnionitis (1–2 in 3000).

Fetal blood sampling:
- Cordocentesis refers to ultrasound guided puncture of umbilical cord (umbilical vein), for either diagnostic (fetal blood sampling) or therapeutic (intrauterine transfusion or drug instillation) purposes performed beyond 18^{+0} completed weeks of gestation using 20–22 G needle under continuous ultrasound guidance.
- Fetal blood can be sampled transabdominally under USG guidance either from the placental cord insertion site, fetal portal vein or a free loop of cord.
- Fetal blood sampling is specially indicated in fetus at higher risk for hematological disorders (quantification of fetal anemia or platelet/lymphocyte count), hydrops and placental mosaicism.
- The risk of fetal loss is between 1 and 2%.

Genetic tests that can be done from the sample obtained is summarized in **Table 8**.

Q11. What are special considerations in invasive testing?

Draft recommendation and evidence:

Role of maternal high risk factors: It is not conclusively proven that risk of fetal loss increases with maternal/uterine high risk factors such as fibroids; Müllerian malformations; chorioamniotic separation; retrochorionic hematoma; previous or current maternal bleeding; maternal body mass index >40 kg/m^2; multiparity (>3 births); manifest vaginal infection; history of three or more miscarriage.

Role of Rh prophylaxis: A prophylactic dose of anti-D immunoglobulin should be administered to all Rh negative, ICT negative women within 72 h postprocedure. A dose of 150 µg is usually recommended when procedures are performed at <20 weeks of gestation.

TABLE 8: Tests that can be performed on a fetal sample.

Test	***Method***	***Turnaround time***	***Advantage***	***Limitation***
Fluorescent in situ hybridization (FISH)	Fluorescent probe for certain chromosomes/ suspected deletions used	24–48 hours	• Rapid • Does not require cell culture or metaphase cells • Can detect mosaicism	• Labor-intensive • Does not test all chromosomes • Cannot detect structural rearrangements
Quantitative fluorescent polymerase chain reaction (qf-PCR)	PCR using markers for certain chromosomes, read on an electrophoretogram	24–48 hours	• Rapid • Automated (less labor-intensive)	• Does not test all chromosomes, • Cannot detect structural rearrangements
Karyotype	Cell culture, followed by analysis of chromosomes on metaphase cells by G-banding	10–14 days	• Shows all chromosomes, including structural rearrangements and large deletions • Can detect mosaicisms	Culture dependent, long turnaround time, labor-intensive
Chromosomal Microarray	Detects gain or loss of genetic material by comparing with standard template. Depending on depth of reading, different arrays can be tested	7–10 days	Submicroscopic changes in chromosomes can be detected depending on depth, algorithm-based	• Cannot detect structural rearrangements • Variants of uncertain significance
Sanger sequencing	Tests single gene with a known sequence	7–10 days	Cost effective, especially if the pathogenic variant is known and the gene is sequenced	Tests only for specific genes or a gene panel

Contd...

Contd…

Test	***Method***	***Turnaround time***	***Advantage***	***Limitation***
Multiplex ligation-dependent probe amplification (MLPA)	Tests variations in copy number of multiple genes, used for detection of deletions and duplications	3–7 days	• Can detect variants in multiple genes responsible for similar phenotype, e.g., Duchenne muscular dystrophy, spinal muscular atrophy • More cost-effective than Sanger sequencing	• May not be able to detect loss of heterozygosity • May show problems in mosaicism
Clinical exome sequencing	Sequences the protein coding regions of disease-causing genes	10–28 days	Can detect variants in multiple genes, correlation with phenotype gives relevant results	• Variants of uncertain significance • Should be interpreted with caution • May detect pathogenic variants with late expressivity
Whole exome sequencing	Sequences the protein coding regions of more than 20,000 genes (~1–2% of genome)	10–28 days	Can detect variants in multiple genes, correlation with phenotype gives relevant results	• Variants of uncertain significance, • Should be interpreted with caution • May detect pathogenic variants with late expressivity
Trio exome sequencing	Sequences the exome of the parents and the proband	10–28 days	Can detect variants in multiple genes, correlation with phenotype gives relevant results. More cost- and time-effective than exome of only proband	• Variants of uncertain significance • Should be interpreted with caution • May detect pathogenic variants with late expressivity
Whole genome sequencing	Sequences the whole genome, including the coding and noncoding regions	10–28 days	Can detect variants in multiple genes, more effective than exome sequencing, correlation with phenotype gives relevant results	• Variants of uncertain significance, • Should be interpreted with caution, • May detect pathogenic variants with late expressivity

Role of antibiotics prophylaxis: Not enough evidence to recommend antibiotic prophylaxis before an invasive procedure routinely.

Role of thromboprophylaxis: There are no available data regarding the discontinuation of thromboprophylaxis before fetal invasive procedures. Regarding prophylactic dosage of aspirin and low-molecular-weight heparin, discontinuation before the procedure does not seem justified clinically. However, withholding a single dose of heparin seems advisable.

Invasive testing in twin gestation: Risk of invasive testing (chorionic villus sampling or amniocentesis) appears to be greater in twins than in singleton pregnancies (2% following chorionic villus sampling and 1.5–2% following amniocentesis).

The risk is similar for transabdominal and transcervical approaches, use of a single-needle or double-needle system, and single or double uterine entry.

Dichorionic twins: Chorionic villus sampling is preferable because it can be performed earlier in gestation. If need arises for selective fetal reduction (due to genetic abnormality) then the chances of miscarriage (risk of loss of the entire pregnancy is significantly lower in the first trimester than in the second trimester (7% vs. 14%)

Monochorionic twins: If monochorionicity has been confirmed before 14 weeks of gestation and the fetuses appear concordant for growth and anatomy, it is acceptable to sample only one amniotic sac. Otherwise, both amniotic sacs should be sampled because of the possibility of rare discordant chromosomal anomalies.

CVS in monochorionic pregnancy may have risk of contamination from the other fetus and hence amniocentesis is preferred.

Limitations of an invasive test:

- Higher risk of cell culture failure with amniocentesis performed in the third trimester. Overall there is a 10% risk of culture failure for third trimester amniocentesis >28 weeks.
- Maternal cell contamination
- Latency time (inherent time required for processing and culture of sample may be of concern depending on gestational age of patient and MTP rules)
- Genetic tests are not mutually exclusive

BIBLIOGRAPHY

1. Agathokleous M, Chaveeva P, Poon LC, et al. Meta-analysis of second-trimester marker for trisomy 21. Ultrasound Obstet Gynecol. 2013;41(3):247-61.
2. American College of Obstetricians and Gynecologists' Committee on Practice Bulletins—Obstetrics; Committee on Genetics; Society for Maternal-Fetal

Medicine. Screening for Fetal Chromosomal Abnormalities: ACOG Practice Bulletin, Number 226. Obstet Gynecol. 2020;136(4):e48-69.

3. Bardi F, Kagan KO, Bilardo CM. First-trimester screening strategies: a balance between costs, efficiency and diagnostic yield. Prenat Diagn. 2023;43(7): 865-72.
4. Boyd PA, Loane M, Garne E, et al. Sex chromosome trisomies in Europe: prevalence, prenatal detection and outcome of pregnancy. Eur J Hum Genet. 2011;19:231-4.
5. Carlson LM, Neeta LV. Prenatal diagnosis: screening and diagnostic tools. Obstet Gynecol Clin North Am. 2017;44(2):245-56.
6. Creasy RK, Resnik R, Iams JD, et al. Prenatal diagnosis of congenital disorders. In: Lockwood CJ, Moore T, Resnik R (Eds). Creasy and Resnik's Maternal-Fetal Medicine: Principles and Practice, 7th edition. Philadelphia: Elsevier; 2014. pp. 417-64.
7. De Domenico R, Faraci M, Hyseni E, et al. Increased nuchal traslucency in normal karyotype fetuses. J Prenat Med. 2011;5(2):23-6.
8. Driscoll DA, Gross SJ; Professional Practice and Guidelines Committee. First trimester diagnosis and screening for fetal aneuploidy. Genet Med. 2008; 10(1):73-5.
9. Driscoll DA, Gross SJ; Professional Practice Guidelines Committee. Screening for fetal aneuploidy and neural tube defects. Genet Med. 2009;11(11):818-21.
10. FIGO Working Group on Good Clinical Practice in Maternal–Fetal Medicine. Good clinical practice advice: Management of twin pregnancy. Int J Gynecol Obstet. 2019;144(3):330-7.
11. Fontoura Oliveira A, Torrão MM, Nogueira R, et al. Recurrent fetal triploidy: is there a genetic cause? BMJ Case Rep. 2021;14:e239843.
12. Forabosco A, Percesepe A, Santucci S. Incidence of non-age-dependent chromosomal abnormalities: a population-based study on 88965 amniocenteses. Eur J Hum Genet. 2009;17:897-903.
13. Genetic Alliance; District of Columbia Department of Health. Understanding Genetics: A District of Columbia Guide for Patients and Health Professionals. Washington (DC): Genetic Alliance; 2010.
14. Ghi T, Sotiriadis A, Calda P, et al. ISUOG Practice Guidelines: invasive procedures for prenatal diagnosis. Ultrasound Obstet Gynecol. 2016;48(2):256-68.
15. Hopkins MK, Dugoff L. Screening for aneuploidy in twins. Am J Obstet Gynecol MFM. 2022;4(2s):100499.
16. Iliescu D, Tudorache S, Comanescu P, et al. Improved detection rate of structural abnormalities in the first trimester using an extended examination protocol. Ultrasound Obstet Gynecol. 2013;42:300-9.
17. Kagan KO, Valencia C, Livanos P, et al. Tricuspid regurgitation in screening for trisomies 21, 18 and 13 and Turner syndrome at 11+0 to 13+6 weeks of gestation. Ultrasound Obstet Gynecol. 2009;33(1):18-22.
18. Khalil A, Rodgers M, Baschat A, et al. ISUOG Practice Guidelines: role of ultrasound in twin pregnancy. Ultrasound Obstet Gynecol. 2016;47(2):247-63.
19. LeFevre NM, Sundermeyer RL. Fetal aneuploidy: screening and diagnostic testing. Am Fam Physician. 2020;101(8):481-8.
20. Li SW, Barrett AN, Gole L, et al. The assessment of combined first trimester screening in women of advanced maternal age in an Asian cohort. Singapore Med J. 2015;56(1):47-52.

21. Li SW, Barrett AN, Gole L, et al. The assessment of combined first trimester screening in women of advanced maternal age in an Asian cohort. Singapore Med J. 2015;56(1):47-52.
22. National Collaborating Center for Women's and Children's Health (UK). Multiple Pregnancy. The Management of Twin and Triplet Pregnancies in the Antenatal Period. Commissioned by the National Institute for Clinical Excellence. London: RCOG Press; 2011.
23. Nicolaides KH. Screening for chromosomal defects. Ultrasound Obstet Gynecol. 2003;21(4):313-21.
24. Nicolaides KH. Screening for fetal aneuploidies at 11 to 13 weeks. Prenat Diagn. 2011;31(1):7-15.
25. Nicoloides K. The 11–13+6 weeks scan. London: Fetal Medicine Foundation; 2004.
26. Olney RS, Moore CA, Khoury MJ, et al. Chorionic villus sampling and amniocentesis: recommendations for prenatal counseling. MMWR Recomm Rep. 1995;44(RR-9):1-12.
27. Petersen OB, Smith E, Van Opstal D, et al. Nuchal translucency of 3.0-3.4 mm an indication for NIPT or microarray? Cohort analysis and literature review. Acta obstetricia et gynecologica Scandinavica. 2020;99(6):765-74.
28. Prats P, Rodríguez I, Comas C, et al. Systematic review of screening for trisomy 21 in twin pregnancies in first trimester combining nuchal translucency and biochemical markers: a meta-analysis. Prenat Diagn. 2014;34:1077-83.
29. Santorum M, Wright D, Syngelaki A, et al. Accuracy of first-trimester combined test in screening for trisomies 21, 18 and 13. Ultrasound Obstet Gynecol. 2017; 49(6):714-20.
30. Society for Maternal-Fetal Medicine (SMFM) Publications Committee. #36: Prenatal aneuploidy screening using cell-free DNA. Am J Obstet Gynecol. 2015;212(6):711-6.
31. Society for Maternal-Fetal Medicine. (2022). Aneuploidy Screening in Twin pregnancies. [online] Available from https://www.smfm.org/news/aneuploidy-screening-in-twin-pregnancies. [Last accessed November, 2024].
32. Sonek J, Nicolaides K. Additional first-trimester ultrasound markers. Clin Lab Med. 2010;30(3):573-92.
33. Sonek JD. Nasal bone in screening for trisomy 21: defining hypoplasia. Am J Obstet Gynecol. 2007;197:335-6.
34. The Fetal Medicine Foundation. FMF Certification: Nuchal Translucency Scan. [online] Available from https://fetalmedicine.org/fmf-certification-2/nuchal-translucency-scan. [Last accessed November, 2024].
35. Wald NJ, Huttly WJ, Hackshaw AK. Antenatal screening for Down's syndrome with the quadruple test. Lancet. 2003;361(9360):835-6.
36. Witters G, Van Robays J, Willekes C, et al. Trisomy 13, 18, 21, Triploidy and Turner syndrome: the 5T's. Look at the hands. Facts Views Vis Obgyn. 2011;3(1):15-21.

CHAPTER 6

Noninvasive Prenatal Testing Guidelines

Priya Kadam, Angela Devanboo

Q1. Who should be offered NIPT?

Draft recommendations:

- Prenatal genetic screening (serum screening with or without nuchal translucency ultrasound or cell-free DNA screening) options should be discussed and offered to all pregnant patients regardless of maternal age or risk of chromosomal abnormality. After review and discussion, every patient has the right to pursue or decline prenatal genetic screening.
- While discussing prenatal testing options in all pregnancies, NIPT can be offered to all pregnant women *irrespective of maternal and gestational age* as it provides highest sensitivity and specificity.
- Cell-free DNA is the most sensitive and specific screening test for the common fetal aneuploidies. Nevertheless, it has the potential for false-positive and false-negative results. Cell-free DNA testing is not equivalent to diagnostic testing.
- Comprehensive pretest counseling is highly recommended while offering NIPT to pregnant women and should include a discussion of baseline age-dependent risk, the potential for false-negative and false-positive results, the difference between screening and diagnostic tests, sensitivity, specificity and what types of follow-up testing to be expected after a NIPT.
- Patients with a positive screening test result for fetal aneuploidy should undergo genetic counseling and a comprehensive ultrasound evaluation. Diagnostic test should be recommended to confirm the positive results.
- NT above >3–3.5 mm, diagnostic testing (and not NIPT) is recommended.

Summary of evidence: NIPT first became available commercially as a screening test in 2012 and since then international guidelines recommended their use only for pregnant women falling in the high risk category, i.e., 35 years and above and having other high risk indications such as an abnormal serum screening. Over the years, with increasing awareness, and superior test performance, NIPT has been recommended for pregnant women in the low-risk category. The American College of Medical Genetics and Genomics (ACMG) guidelines published in 2022, strongly recommends the use of NIPT over traditional methods for all pregnant women. NIPT can also be offered to pregnant women with clinical indications such as women with advanced maternal age, positive to intermediate risk on conventional serum screening, detection of soft markers on ultrasound, previous history of pregnancy with chromosomal abnormality, family history of chromosomal abnormality and anxious pregnant women. However, invasive prenatal diagnosis is recommended when one or more fetal structural abnormalities are detected on an ultrasound examination as there is a background risk of 6% of clinically relevant deletions or duplications. Specifically for NT measurement, a value >3.5 mm is known to be associated with other abnormalities and an NIPT alone may miss 2–10% of cases with a pathogenic variation. India has a wide range in affordability among patients and in a low to moderate resource setting, the cost benefit analysis mostly leans toward using NIPT as a contingent screening tool in high risk population and also as a primary screening in certain situations.

Research gap: With the falling prices of NIPT there is no clear cost-benefit analysis in the Indian setting which can take into account the costs of different screening strategies, sensitivities, most importantly patient preference and further management options.

Q2. When is the right time to do NIPT?

Draft recommendations:

- NIPT is recommended to be performed after the first trimester NT scan
- A maternal blood sample is obtained ≥10 weeks (with some labs offering testing beginning at 9 weeks) of pregnancy. Usually performed at 11 to 13 weeks.
- If contingent screening is adopted, NIPT can be offered to women with high risk on serum screening.
- If no screening has been performed, NIPT is a good option as it is not gestational age sensitive, technically there is no upper limit on when the test can be performed.

Summary of evidence: Technically, NIPT can be offered any time after 9–10 weeks of gestation (depending on the technology used by the laboratory offering NIPT) as sufficient fetal fraction is expected by then. There are two approaches to the use of NIPT, as a first line screening or as contingent screening. Regardless, an ultrasound, performed prior to NIPT sampling can provide useful information such as viability of fetus, number of fetuses, presence of vanishing twin and any abnormality requiring direct diagnostic testing. Also, unlike maternal serum screening NIPT is not bound by gestational windows. There is no upper limit up to when NIPT can be performed till term.

In India, the NIPT cost is taken care of by the patients and the insurances usually do not cover NIPT expenses. Due to the higher cost of NIPT, the patients prefer to opt for traditional serum screening followed by NIPT in case of increased risk on serum screening. This is called contingent NIPT screening. This method has proven to be cost-effective and beneficial as the number of pregnant women having to undergo an invasive procedure will be significantly reduced.

Research gap: There is not enough Indian literature coverage on the use of various forms of screening tests for aneuploidies, including maternal serum screening as well NIPT in clinical settings, the preference of clinicians and pregnant women. An additional study on awareness of health care providers such as obstetricians, genetic counselors regarding the nuances of aneuploidy screening tests is currently not available.

Q3. What is the sensitivity and specificity of NIPT compared to maternal serum screening?

Draft recommendations:

- NIPT is the most accurate screening test in terms of sensitivity, specificity, positive predictive value and false positive rates for the common autosomal aneuploidies (trisomies 21, 13, and 18) in unselected singleton populations, and those at known increased probability.
- The relative comparison between different screening tests for the parameters mentioned above as well costs should be covered during the pre-test counseling.
- False positive result may occur with NIPT. Therefore, it is strongly recommended that all pregnant individuals with a high risk NIPT result have genetic counseling and diagnostic testing if they are considering termination of pregnancy.

Summary of evidence: Results obtained from NEXT study published by Norton el al., in 2015, who evaluated the performance of cell free DNA (cfDNA) screening and standard screening (nuchal translucency + double marker screening) in unselected population are summarized in the following **Table 1**.

The American College of Obstetricians and Gynecologists (ACOG) guidelines published on "screening for fetal chromosomal abnormalities" in the year 2020 have demonstrated that cfDNA-based test, i.e., NIPT is the most sensitive screening test with sensitivity of 99% for detecting trisomy 21. Similarly, the American College of Medical Genetics and Genomics (ACMG) developed an evidence-based guideline on "noninvasive prenatal screening (NIPS) for fetal chromosome abnormalities in a general-risk population" in the year 2022, which strongly recommends the use of NIPT as a first-line screening test due to its high detection rate and low false positive rate. Based on the chromosomal condition, the detection rates varied, i.e., 98.8% (trisomy 21), 98.83% (trisomy 18), and 92.85% (trisomy 13).

TABLE 1: Performance of standard screening compared to NIPT in unselected population.

Performance metrics	***NIPT***			***Standard screening***		
	Trisomy 21	Trisomy 18	Trisomy 13	Trisomy 21	Trisomy 18	Trisomy 13
Sensitivity	100%	90%	100%	78.9%	80%	50%
Specificity	99.9%	100%	100%	94.6%	99.7%	99.7%
Positive predictive value	80.9%	90%	50%	3.4%	14%	3.4%

Q4. What is the optimum fetal fraction requirement for NIPT?

Draft recommendations:

- The percentage of fetal DNA found in maternal blood is known as the fetal fraction. Typical range is 3–13% of maternal cfDNA.
- Fetal fraction is a critical quality metric and clinicians should be aware of minimum fetal fraction from various test providers. Substantial variation exists between laboratories and test methodologies. Laboratories should perform their own internal validation of their limit of detection and threshold for "no call" results.
- The fetal fraction is critical to the success of NIPT. Minimum required approximately 2–4%. Sensitivity drops with lower fetal fraction and if too low, test failure will result.
- The possibility of a repeat sample in case the fetal fraction falls below the threshold for reporting should be discussed with the patients before offering NIPT.

Summary of evidence: Fetal fraction refers to the proportion of cfDNA fragments in maternal plasma that arise from the placenta as a percentage of the total cfDNA. The fetal fraction sees a relatively wide distribution and is affected by factors such as gestational age, maternal weight, maternal race, fetal karyotype, and maternal medical conditions. Fetal fraction is an important quality metric.

The minimum fetal fraction required for reporting results on NIPT ranges between 2% and 4%. The fetal fraction threshold depends on the technology being used. Fiorentino F, 2016, conducted a study to understand the limit of detection and the performance of NIPT at lower fetal fraction. This study concluded that the limit of detection should be based on the specific NIPT technology being employed and not fixed at 4%. Out of 105 pregnancies with confirmed chromosomal abnormality, 25 of them had fetal fraction between 2% and 4% on NIPT. If the cut off of 4% was fixed, the diagnosis for these

25 pregnancies would have been delayed. Furthermore, Borth H, illustrated that the negative predictive value remained high, i.e., 98.1% for cases with fetal fraction less than 4%. In the Indian population, the mean fetal fraction observed was 8.3%. Some reports indicate that repeated low fetal fraction is associated with aneuploidy.

Q5. What is the next course of action if NIPT gives a no-call result?

Draft recommendations:

- The clinician should be aware of the possible reasons for no-call NIPT results and the patient should be explained in the pre-test counseling.
- Inform patients that there is an increased risk of aneuploidy.
- Offer genetic counseling, detailed ultrasound evaluation and diagnostic testing.
- Repeat screening "may be considered" with a success rate 75–80% (less with high BMI)
- Decisions for diagnostic testing (and not repeat screening) should be considered in cases where the gestational age is advanced and further delay may complicate access to reproductive options or there is a fetal abnormality noted on ultrasound scan.

Summary of evidence: A repeat sample may be suggested for various factors, both pre- and postanalytical factors. The preanalytical factors include low sample volume, wrong sample collection tube, and lysed sample. The post analytical factors mostly include fetal fraction falls below the threshold and quality control failures. When the fetal fraction falls below the required cut off, a "no-call result" is reported and a repeat sample collection may be requested. About 1% of initial samples may give a no-call result. The most common reason for a no call result is low fetal fraction, other biological factors have been identified to influence the fetal fraction such as maternal factors that include maternal weight, maternal medical condition (autoimmune disease), and medications (low molecular weight heparin). Fetal-Placental factors include gestational age, crown rump length, fetal aneuploidy and multiple gestations. A repeat testing provides a result approximately 75–80% of the time as it will invariably be performed at a later gestational age. It is a general consensus that insufficient fetal fraction, carries an increased risk for fetal aneuploidy, particularly for trisomy 18 and trisomy 13. About 4.7–>17% of aneuploidy rates have been associated with insufficient fetal fraction failures. Caldwell S, 2021, demonstrated that insufficient fetal fraction was not an indicator of aneuploidy risk or adverse pregnancy outcomes. In this study, 109 patients had repeated low fetal fraction on NIPT and 76 patients with known birth outcomes resulted in apparently healthy liveborns. Therefore, a repeat NIPT can be considered as a next step in cases of "no-call result". Depending on the gestational age and the maternal weight, a repeat sample can be offered to the pregnant women. The background risk, detailed ultrasound and patient preferences should be considered before arranging for a resampling for NIPT. The women should also be made aware of the possibility of increased risk of fetal abnormality in case of repeated NIPT failures. Diagnostic testing should be recommended if a fetal abnormality is detected on ultrasound.

Q6. Should all high risk results be confirmed on invasive testing?

Draft recommendations:

- Principles of informed choice should be maintained in the face of "routinization" of prenatal screening and the expanded scope of some NIPT assays.
- Post-test counseling should be offered to pregnant women regarding the implications of high-risk NIPT results. Those with a high risk NIPT result should be offered diagnostic testing for confirmation.

Summary of evidence: NIPT has established itself as a superior screening test with high sensitivity and specificity for screening common chromosomal abnormalities. As illustrated in **Table 1**, the cell-free DNA-based test offers high positive predictive value when compared to standard screening methods. However, the test should not be considered as an alternative for prenatal diagnostic test. False-positive results can occur on NIPT. Certain biological factors such as confined placental mosaicism, vanishing twin, maternal mosaicism or underlying maternal malignancy can influence the cell-free DNA based test. Confined placental mosaicism can occur in 1–2% of pregnancies. Certain conditions like trisomy 13 and monosomy X have high risks of placental mosaicism and amniocentesis may be preferred over chorionic villus sampling in cases where no fetal anomalies are detected on an ultrasound. Therefore, patients with high-risk NIPT results must undergo genetic counseling and the possibility of false positive result on NIPT should be explained. Comprehensive ultrasound and diagnostic testing should be recommended and must be performed before considering the option of terminating the pregnancy.

Q7. What is the sensitivity of NIPT in twin pregnancies? Higher order pregnancies?

Draft recommendations:

- *Cell-free DNA screening can be performed in twin pregnancies.* Overall, performance of screening for trisomy 21 by cell-free DNA in twin pregnancies is encouraging, but the total number of reported affected cases is small. Given the small number of affected cases it is difficult to determine an accurate detection rate for trisomy 18 and 13.
- High risk NIPT results should be followed by diagnostic testing performed on both the fetuses before taking any irreversible clinical decisions.

Summary of evidence: With high performance of NIPT in screening singleton pregnancies, the performance of NIPT in twin pregnancies has also been evaluated. The meta-analysis study carried out by He Y, 2020 consisting of overall 25 studies assessed the performance of NIPT in twin pregnancies. This study revealed a positive predictive value (PPV) of 98.99% and negative predictive value (NPV) of 99.58% for trisomy 21, PPV - 87.93% and NPV - 99.95% for trisomy 18 and PPV - 78.57% and NPV - 99.88% for trisomy 13.

ISPD Position Statement on cfDNA screening in multiple pregnancies published in 2020, recommends the use of NIPT as a screening test in twin pregnancies. The guidelines indicate that the detection rates for detecting trisomy 21, trisomy 18 and trisomy 13 were 98.8%, 93.1%, and 75% for twin gestations. They also remark on the high predictive value compared to the conventional serum screening. ACMG 2022 also endorses the use of NIPT over traditional screening techniques in screening fetal aneuploidy in the fetus. Currently, most of the laboratories offering NIPT for twins have limited to screening only common trisomies (trisomies 21, 18, and 13). Based on the NIPT technology used, screening for monosomy X can be offered for twins. Currently, SNP-based NIPT can screen for monosomy X and can only be offered in monozygotic twin pregnancies. As with singleton pregnancies, fetal fraction (FF) is a critical parameter for NIPT in screening twin pregnancies as well. The test failures due to insufficient FF are high in twin pregnancies as compared to singleton. The no call rate ranged between 1.6% and 13.2% in twin pregnancies. While there is no minimum fetal fraction requirement for twin pregnancies, the threshold is set in such a way that the overall fetal fraction obtained is twice as that of singleton pregnancies. Twin pregnancies with high risk results on NIPT screening, should be offered genetic counseling followed by comprehensive ultrasound evaluation and prenatal diagnosis for both the fetuses.

Research gap: Currently, the data on the clinical utility of NIPT in triplet pregnancies is sparse. The professional guidelines do not recommend nor comment on the use of NIPT as a screening test for higher-order gestations.

Q8. Can NIPT be offered for pregnancies with a history of vanishing twins?

Draft recommendations:

- In multifetal gestations, if a fetal demise, vanishing twin, or anomaly is identified in one fetus, there is a significant risk of an inaccurate test result if serum-based aneuploidy screening or cell-free DNA is used. This information should be reviewed with the patient and diagnostic testing should be offered.
- NIPT can be offered with care in pregnant women with a history of vanishing twins.

- Presence of the vanishing twin should be communicated to the laboratory.
- Sample collection should be performed with as long a gap as possible after fetal demise.
- Results should be interpreted by the clinician with care.
- Possibility of a false positive in case of high risk NIPT should be conveyed to the couple.

Summary of evidence: There is a higher possibility of false positive and discordant results when a vanishing twin is present. There is no clear data on how long the DNA from the vanished twin is present in maternal circulation and can potentially confound the result; it is shown to still be present even after 8 weeks after fetal demise. In a study of 206 vanishing twin pregnancies, the VT pregnancies exhibited a higher prevalence of screen-positive cases (5.8% vs. 2.5%), and false positive rates (FPR) (2.6% vs. 0.3%) than singleton pregnancies. The same study indicated that these discrepancies lower when the test is performed after 14 weeks. In a systematic review of NIPT performance with a history of known vanishing twins, aneuploidies were systematically detected but the positive predictive value was lower as compared to pure singleton pregnancies. Though the American College of Obstetricians and Gynecologists states that NIPS should not be performed in such circumstances, the recent ACMG practice guidelines say that there is no evidence to support avoiding NIPT in pregnant women with a history of vanishing twin but the patient should be counseled that accuracy can be impacted.

Q9. Should NIPT be offered to screen for microdeletions? What are rare autosomal aneuploidies?

Draft recommendations:

- NIPT can be offered to pregnant women for 22q11.2 microdeletion syndrome. The other microdeletion syndromes show a low positive predictive value and therefore may still be at the discretion of the clinicians.
- There is insufficient data to assess the performance and clinical utility of routine NIPT for rare autosomal aneuploidies (RAT).
- Insufficient evidence to screen for other duplications/deletions but there are "families for whom NIPT for CNVs could be offered based on the pregnancy or family history".
- Appropriate pre-test counseling should be offered for patients who opt screening for microdeletions and rare autosomal aneuploidies on NIPT.
- The discretion of sending NIPT for rare autosomal aneuploidies is the choice of the clinician and patient preference. Sometimes, it can provide an explanation for IUGR, fetal demise and congenital anomalies.
- RAT is therefore not recommended for the routine care of unselected populations.

- Where screening for RATs is performed, management after a high chance result requires expert post-test counseling and specialist management.
- Due to the high likelihood of Confined placental mosaicism underlying a positive NIPT result for a RAT, amniocentesis is the single most informative test for fetal karyotype.
- If NIPT returns as high-chance result for a trisomy involving an imprinted chromosome, amniocentesis with appropriate studies to detect UPD is recommended.

Summary of evidence: The current NIPT providers offer NIPT for predominantly screening common microdeletions such as 22q11.2 deletion syndrome or DiGeorge syndrome (DGS), 1p36 deletion syndrome, Cri-du-chat syndrome, Prader–Willi syndrome, Angelman syndrome, and other rarer microdeletions. Based on the technology and the syndrome the positive predictive value (PPV) varies for screening these conditions. Among these, DGS has the highest PPV (16–93%) whereas for others, the PPV can range from 0–75%. Till 2023 no international guidelines recommended NIPT for microdeletion syndromes due to insufficient data but ACMG in 2023 has recommended the conditional use of NIPT of 22q11.2 microdeletion syndrome as there is moderate evidence and incidence is sufficiently high.

According to Benn et al. (2019), the most likely pregnancy outcome for a positive RAT pregnancy is a normal live birth in ~50% of the cases while other 50% has adverse pregnancy outcomes such as miscarriage, structural as well as genetic abnormalities, neurodevelopmental delay, true fetal mosaicism, fetal growth restriction and preterm delivery, uniparental disomy but the outcome was dependent on the specific RAT and gestational age at the time of testing.

Q10. What are the possible incidental findings that can be detected on NIPT? Should these be reported to the referring clinician and/or the patients?

Draft recommendations:

- Positive NIPT results should be investigated further.
- Because of the methodology of NIPS, there is the potential to incidentally identify certain maternal conditions. This includes the identification of maternal chromosome imbalances and unsuspected maternal malignancies. The possibilities of identification of maternal abnormalities, though rare should be incorporated in the pre-test counseling.
- Detection of multiple aneuploidies on NIPT, warrants further investigation in the mother as well.

Summary of evidence: False positives on NIPT have been attributed to different biological factors including maternal factors such as mosaicism or copy number variations. NIPT screening for sex chromosomal aneuploidy (SCA) can reveal a previously unknown maternal genetic abnormality. Therefore, the analysis while reporting SCA on NIPT should be carried out cautiously and the results should in interpreted carefully. For example, positive risk for Monosomy X on NIPT should be investigated further as the age-related risk of monosomy X mosaicism in the lymphocytes of the pregnant women can confound the result for the fetus.

The positive predictive value for detecting maternal malignancy on NIPT ranges between 7.6% and 73.3%. The type of cancers detected based on NIPT findings are lymphoma, breast cancer, colorectal cancer, liver cancer, gynecological cancer, leukemia, multiple myeloma, and lung cancer. Currently, there are no scientific guidelines discussing possible detection of maternal malignancy on NIPT. ACOG, 2020 recommends that in cases where multiple aneuploidies are detected the pregnant woman should be offered a physical examination (lymphadenopathy, breast, and thyroid masses), complete blood count, complete metabolic profile, Pap test, and fecal occult blood testing in cases where there is a high suspicion of malignancy. ACOG, 2020 also recommends that the pre-test counseling includes the topic of the possibility of incidental findings that might reveal a maternal condition.

Q11. What are the topics that should be discussed during pre-test and post-test counseling while offering NIPT?

Draft recommendations:

- Patients should be informed that NIPT is a screening test and negative results do not eliminate the possibility of a fetal abnormality.
- Comprehensive pre-test counseling is highly recommended while offering NIPT to pregnant women as sensitivity, specificity, positive predictive value and false positive rate need to be covered during pre-test counseling. Clinicians should ensure that pre-test counseling promotes patient autonomy whilst providing a supportive environment for shared discussion and decision making in line with the patient's values.
- Post-test counseling for those with low chance results should include a caveat that NIPT does not exclude all genetic conditions and that false-negative results may occur.
- Individuals with a high chance result should also be informed that FPR may occur, and that diagnostic testing is recommended prior to management decisions, particularly if termination of pregnancy is being considered. When a high chance result is discussed with a patient, clinicians should ensure they present an informed description of the suspected condition, including discussion about the range of phenotypic variation. Further, they should provide educational materials that are developed in conjunction with advocacy organizations and consider offering a referral to a health care professional with expertise on that condition.

- Where NIPT has uncovered incidental findings relevant to maternal health, referral to a genetics specialist is recommended to ensure appropriate management of that parent and any other relevant family members.

BIBLIOGRAPHY

1. American College of Obstetricians and Gynecologists' Committee on Practice Bulletins—Obstetrics; Committee on Genetics; Society for Maternal-Fetal Medicine. Screening for Fetal Chromosomal Abnormalities: ACOG Practice Bulletin, Number 226. Obstet Gynecol. 2020;136(4):e48-69.
2. Balaguer N, Mateu-Brull E, Serra V, et al. Should vanishing twin pregnancies be systematically excluded from cell-free fetal DNA testing? Prenat Diagn. 2021;41(10):1241-8.
3. Benn P, Malvestiti F, Grimi B, et al. Rare autosomal trisomies: comparison of detection through cell-free DNA analysis and direct chromosome preparation of chorionic villus samples. Ultrasound Obstet Gynecol. 2019;54(4):458-67.
4. Benn P, Rebarber A. Non-invasive prenatal testing in the management of twin pregnancies. Prenat Diagn. 2021;41(10):1233-40.
5. Borth H, Teubert A, Glaubitz R, et al. Analysis of cell-free DNA in a consecutive series of 13,607 routine cases for the detection of fetal chromosomal aneuploidies in a single center in Germany. Arch Gynecol Obstet. 2021;303:1407-14.
6. Caldwell S, Almasri E, Schmidt L, et al. Not all low fetal fraction cell-free DNA screening failures are at increased risk for aneuploidy. Prenat Diagn. 2021; 41(11):1372-9.
7. Curnow KJ, Wilkins-Haug L, Ryan A, et al. Detection of triploid, molar, and vanishing twin pregnancies by a single-nucleotide polymorphism based noninvasive prenatal test. Am J Obstet Gynecol. 2015;212:79.e1-9.
8. Devanboo A, Nathan DC, Mahalingam SK, et al. Detection of 22q11.2 deletion syndrome by single-nucleotide polymorphism based non-invasive prenatal test. Indian J Obstet Gynecol Res. 2023;10(3):374-8.
9. Dondorp W, De Wert G, Bombard Y, et al. Non-invasive prenatal testing for aneuploidy and beyond: challenges of responsible innovation in prenatal screening. Eur J Hum Genet. 2015;23(11):1438-50.
10. Dungan JS, Klugman S, Darilek S, et al.; ACMG Board of Directors. Noninvasive prenatal screening (NIPS) for fetal chromosome abnormalities in a general-risk population: an evidence-based clinical guideline of the American College of Medical Genetics and Genomics (ACMG). Genet Med. 2023;25(2):100336.
11. Fiorentino F, Bono S, Pizzuti F, et al. The importance of determining the limit of detection of non-invasive prenatal testing methods. Prenat Diagn. 2016;36(4):304-11.
12. Gromminger S, Yagmur E, Erkan S, et al. Fetal aneuploidy detection by cell-free DNA sequencing for multiple pregnancies and quality issues with vanishing twins. J Clin Med. 2014;3(3):679-92.
13. He Y, Wang Y, Li Z, et al. Clinical performance of non-invasive prenatal testing for trisomies 21, 18 and 13 in twin pregnancies: a cohort study and a systematic meta-analysis. Acta Obstet Gynecol Scand. 2020;99:731-43.

14. Hui L, Bianchi DW. Fetal fraction and noninvasive prenatal testing: what clinicians need to know. Prenat Diagn. 2020;40(2):155-63.
15. Hui L, Ellis K, Mayen D, et al. Position statement from the International Society for Prenatal Diagnosis on the use of non-invasive prenatal testing for the detection of fetal chromosomal conditions in singleton pregnancies. Prenat Diagn. 2023;43(7):814-28.
16. Lenaerts L, Che H, Brison N, et al. Breast cancer detection and treatment monitoring using a noninvasive prenatal testing platform: utility in pregnant and nonpregnant populations. Clin Chem. 2020;66(11):1414-23.
17. Lenaerts L, Theunis M, Amant F, et al. Non-invasive prenatal testing: when results suggests maternal cancer. Med Genet. 2023;35(4):285-95.
18. Liang D, Cram DS, Tan HU, et al. Clinical utility of noninvasive prenatal screening for expanded chromosome disease syndromes. Genet Med. 2019; 21(9):1998-2006.
19. Lin Y, Liang D, Wang Y, et al. Analyzing false-negative results detected in low-risk non-invasive prenatal screening cases. Mol Genet Genomic Med. 2020;8: e1185.
20. Mahalingam S, Devanboo A, Pradhan A, et al. True fetal trisomy 22 detected using genome-wide noninvasive prenatal testing. J Obstet Gynaecol India. 2023; 73(2):180-2.
21. Massa JD, Arora V, Lallar M, Current status of noninvasive prenatal testing and counselling considerations: an Indian perspective. J Fetal Med. 2020;7(1): 9-16.
22. Norton ME, Jacobsson B, Swamy GK, et al. Cell-free DNA analysis for noninvasive examination of trisomy. N Engl J Med. 2015;372(17):1589-97.
23. Palomaki GE, Chiu RWK, Pertile MD, et al. International Society for Prenatal Diagnosis Position Statement: cell free (cf) DNA screening for Down syndrome in multiple pregnancies. Prenat Diagn. 2021;41(10):1222-32.
24. Pertile MD, Halks-Miller M, Flowers N, et al. Rare autosomal trisomies, revealed by maternal plasma DNA sequencing, suggest increased risk of feto-placental disease. Sci Transl Med. 2017;9:eaan1240.
25. Seong JS, Han YJ, Kim MH, et al. The risk of preterm birth in vanishing twin: a multicenter prospective cohort study. PloS One. 2020;15(5):e0233097.
26. Shao L, Akkari Y, Cooley LD, et al.; ACMG Laboratory Quality Assurance Committee Chromosomal microarray analysis, including constitutional and neoplastic disease applications, 2021 revision: a technical standard of the American College of Medical Genetics and Genomics (ACMG). Genet Med. 2021;23(10):1818-29.
27. Srebniak MI, de Wit MC, Diderich KE, et al. Enlarged NT (≥3.5 mm) in the first trimester—not all chromosome aberrations can be detected by NIPT. Mol Cytogenet. 2016;9(1):69.
28. Taylor JB, Chock VY, Hudgins L. NIPT in a clinical setting: an analysis of uptake in the first months of clinical availability. J Genet Couns. 2014;23(1):72-8.
29. van der Meij KRM, Sistermans EA, Macville MVE, et al. TRIDENT-2: national implementation of genome-wide non-invasive prenatal testing as a first-tier screening test in the Netherlands. Am J Hum Genet. 2019;105(6):1091-101.
30. van Eekhout JCA, Bekker MN, Bax CJ, et al. Non-invasive prenatal testing (NIPT) in twin pregnancies affected by early single fetal demise: A systematic review of NIPT and vanishing twins. Prenat Diagn. 2023;43(7):829-37.

31. Verma IC, Dua-Puri R, Bijarnia-Mahay S. ACMG 2016 Update on Noninvasive Prenatal Testing for Fetal Aneuploidy: Implications for India. J Fetal Med. 2017;4:1-6.
32. Verma IC, Puri R, Venkataswamy E, et al. Single nucleotide polymorphism-based noninvasive prenatal testing: experience in India. J Obstet Gynecol India. 2018;68:462-70.
33. Wapner RJ, Babiarz JE, Levy B, et al. Expanding the scope of noninvasive prenatal testing: detection of fetal microdeletion syndromes. Am J Obstet Gynecol. 2015;212:332.e1-9.
34. Wapner RJ, Martin CL, Levy B, et al. Chromosomal microarray versus karyotyping for prenatal diagnosis. N Engl J Med. 2012;367(23):2175-84.

CHAPTER 7

Prenatal Genetic Evaluation of Fetal Anomalies

Shagun Aggarwal

Q1. Is genetic workup needed for prenatally detected anomalies?

Draft recommendations: All prenatally detected fetal anomalies should undergo genetic evaluation to ascertain the possibility of an underlying syndrome.

Summary of evidence: Structural anomalies detected in the prenatal period have a high probability of being part of a genetic syndrome. Studies have revealed that numerical chromosomal disorders can be seen in up to 30%, microdeletions/microduplications in 6–10% and single gene disorders in 20–30% of such cases. If an anomaly is due to a genetic syndrome, the prognosis of the fetus is guarded as compared to an isolated anomaly, as postnatally additional functional impairments like intellectual disability are likely. Genetic evaluation helps in ascertaining whether the anomaly is truly isolated, in which case the outcome would depend on the anomaly per se versus anomaly being part of a genetic syndrome; and this aids in appropriate counseling, prognostication, and management plan for the families.

Q2. Should the genetic workup be a noninvasive screening test or an invasive diagnostic test?

Draft recommendations: An invasive diagnostic test by chorionic villus sampling (11–14 weeks) or amniocentesis (after 16 weeks) should be performed in case of an anomaly* is detected on prenatal imaging.

*Anomaly for the purpose of this guideline includes a structural malformation, other major morphological abnormality in the fetus like nonimmune hydrops fetalis, arthrogryposis, skeletal dysplasia, etc., and evolving/dynamic abnormalities like ventriculomegaly, club feet, single cavity effusions, etc. Some isolated anomalies such as gastroschisis, posterior urethral valves, congenital pulmonary airway malformation, and amniotic band may not require genetic evaluation provided the ultrasound has been performed by a highly skilled operator and no diagnostic dilemmas exist.

Summary of evidence: The risk of an underlying genetic syndrome in cases of fetal anomalies is high, thereby placing the pregnancy in the high risk category. As screening tests are designed to screen the high risk cases from amongst all pregnancies, such tests have limited sensitivity and specificity. Also, screening tests are primarily targeted toward common chromosomal abnormalities involving chromosomes 21, 13, and 18, and these cannot provide information regarding single gene disorders or microdeletions/

microduplication syndromes. Hence, in a pregnancy already at high risk of being affected with a genetic syndrome due to fetal anomaly, there is no role of a screening test. Such pregnancies need to undergo invasive sampling either by chorionic villus sampling in first trimester or amniocentesis in second trimester. Sample obtained by these procedures can be used for diagnostic genetic testing to provide definitive information regarding the fetus. Some fetal anomalies like gastroschisis, posterior urethral valves, congenital pulmonary airway malformation, amniotic band, etc., have not been shown to have a genetic association. Invasive fetal sampling maybe avoided in such instances. However, as these can mimic other anomalies of genetic origin or may not be truly isolated, unless the ultrasound has been done by highly skilled operator and the diagnosis established beyond reasonable doubt, a genetic testing or screening test maybe considered in such scenarios too.

Q3. What information should be obtained by the obstetrician before ordering a genetic test?

Draft recommendations: An obstetrician should obtain a three-generation family history with attention to similarly affected family members, bad obstetric history, consanguinity and other case based specific details. History of teratogen exposure and maternal diseases which may have a role in causation of the fetal anomaly needs to be assessed.

Summary of evidence: Eliciting a three-generation family history, preferably in form of a pedigree chart helps in recognizing inherited nature of the fetal anomaly and the likely inheritance pattern. Such a history should include leading queries regarding similar or overlapping anomalies in previous offsprings, parents (who may have undergone a surgical intervention and are presently asymptomatic) as well as extended family. This helps in providing clues toward probable genetic etiology and chose a genetic test accordingly. In addition, history of consanguinity, bad obstetric history, intellectual disability, childhood onset chronic illnesses like neuromuscular disorders, short stature, etc., and confirmed genetic disorders should be elicited. These may provide clues regarding possible genetic etiology of the anomaly detected in the current pregnancy. Various teratogens or maternal conditions may result in fetal anomalies, and these need to be ascertained by careful history. Some of the examples are maternal diabetes associated neural tube defect, caudal regression, focal femoral hypoplasia, etc., fetal phenytoin syndrome, fetal warfarin syndrome, and many others. Similarly, some genetic diseases in the mother may be missed and may be causative of fetal anomaly, e.g., maternal myotonic dystrophy resulting in fetal joint deformities, maternal phenylketonuria resulting in microcephaly and many others.

Q4. Which genetic test should be performed on the fetal sample?

Draft recommendations: Comprehensive genetic evaluation should be done comprising of chromosomal microarray with or without rapid aneuploidy testing for common chromosomal abnormalities and exome sequencing (ES) for single gene disorders. Choice of genetic test can be individualized on a case to case basis and guided by type of anomaly, pattern of anomalies and family history. Maternal cell contamination needs to be tested for all invasive fetal samples. Trio versus solo fetal exome can be discussed on a case to case basis.

Summary of evidence: In view of significant contribution of chromosomal disorders and microdeletion/microduplication syndrome to fetal anomalies, international guidelines by various professional societies recommend chromosomal microarray (CMA) as the test of choice on the fetal sample. This test is able to detect all numerical chromosomal abnormalities as well as submicroscopic microdeletions and microduplications which are missed by karyotype. In some instances, a rapid aneuploidy test like QF-PCR, FISH, or MLPA for five chromosomes (13, 18, 21, X, and Y) can be done in conjunction with CMA, especially if period of gestation is advanced. These tests provide information regarding common chromosomal abnormalities in 24–48 hours. Also, in special circumstances like pattern of anomalies fitting a specific genetic syndrome, family pedigree indicating a single gene disorder, phenotypes like skeletal dysplasia, arthrogryposis, nonimmune hydrops, etc. Exome sequencing should be considered as a first tier test along with chromosomal microarray as these scenarios indicate a high risk of fetus being affected with a single gene disorder. Emerging evidence indicates that 20–30% of fetal anomalies are due to a single gene disorder. Hence, exome sequencing should be considered as a second tier test once CMA is normal for all anomalies. Trio exome sequencing which involves parallel ES for fetus and couple is useful for detection of de novo variants and phasing of variants for autosomal recessive disorders. This helps in reducing turnaround time, but is associated with increase in cost. Maternal cell contamination study by suitable molecular assays is mandatory for all prenatal samples, as contamination of fetal sample by maternal cells causes erroneous results.

Q5. Is there a difference in genetic test in case of lethal versus nonlethal anomalies?

Draft recommendations: Both lethal and nonlethal anomalies need a genetic evaluation as mentioned earlier. In addition, in case of lethal anomaly, a perinatal autopsy needs to be performed for detailed phenotypic delineation.

Summary of evidence: The contribution of genetic syndromes exists in both lethal and non-lethal anomalies. Pregnancy is likely to be carried till term in case of nonlethal anomalies, and comprehensive genetic evaluation is important for accurate prognostication. In case of lethal anomalies, families may choose interruption of pregnancy and may not be willing for a genetic evaluation. However, in cases with a syndromic etiology, there is a risk of recurrence in subsequent conceptions. The magnitude of this risk depends on the underlying genetic disorder, and can range from 1% for free trisomies to 25–50% for various single gene disorders. A perinatal autopsy is important in these scenarios to collect comprehensive phenotypic information regarding the fetus. Various studies show detection of 16–33% additional findings on a perinatal autopsy which changes the counseling and recurrence risk for families. In addition, sample for genetic test needs to be obtained at time of delivery or soon after. Storage of this sample and subsequent workup prior to planning next pregnancy is a reasonable option for families.

Q6. Which fetal samples can be used for genetic testing?

Draft recommendations: Prenatally collected samples such as chorionic villi, amniotic fluid, cord blood, or intrapartum/postnatally collected samples such as cord blood, intracardiac blood, skin, and umbilical cord can be used for genetic testing.

Summary of evidence: Genetic tests like CMA or ES are performed on DNA samples. DNA can be obtained from a variety of fetal samples. Prenatally, samples such as chorionic villi, amniotic fluid, or sometime cord blood can be collected by invasive sampling. During intrapartum period or immediately postdelivery/expulsion, samples such as cord blood, skin biopsy, and umbilical cord segment can be collected for DNA extraction. Blood samples need to be collected in EDTA vials. Tissue samples can be collected in normal saline or RPMI medium. Amniotic fluid samples need to be collected in sterile tubes. These samples should be transported to genetic laboratory at the earliest and once DNA is extracted, it can be stored long term or subjected to genetic tests as per scenario. In case of delay, samples can be stored at 2–4°C for 24–48 hours. Nonviable cells can be used for DNA extraction.

Q7. What information should be provided to the laboratory?

Draft recommendations: The laboratory should be provided detailed information regarding the ultrasound findings, preferably using standard terminology like Human Phenotype Ontology terms as well as information as mentioned in answer to question number 3 as above.

Summary of evidence: Genome wide tests like CMA and ES reveal thousands of variants, only one of which is usually causative of the fetal anomaly. Bioinformatics analysis of such tests and shortlisting of relevant variant requires detailed and clear clinical details. Multiple studies have showed that use of standard terminologies to describe the abnormal phenotypic findings helps the laboratory to generate a meaningful report. One of such standard terminology resource is the Human Phenotype Ontology (HPO). If access to this resource is not possible, a detailed description of the ultrasound findings should be provided to the laboratory. In addition, as the family history provides important clue to the genetic diagnoses, this should be elicited and included in the test request form.

Q8. What pre and post-test counseling should be provided to families?

Draft recommendations: Counseling should preferably be performed by a clinical genetics expert or fetal medicine specialist. Pretest counseling should include information regarding the expected diagnostic yield of the genetic test, anticipated prognosis of a genetic syndrome, risk of invasive sampling, turnaround time and cost; and possibility of detection of a variant of uncertain clinical significance. Post-test counseling for a pathogenic/likely pathogenic variant on the genetic report should include prognostication of the detected disorder. Post-test counseling for a negative genetic report should include reassurance with a mention of residual risk due to test limitations. All cases with variants of uncertain significance should be referred to a clinical geneticist.

Summary of evidence: Genome wide genetic tests are based on complex technologies and interpretation of the huge amount of data obtained from these tests is a complicated process and depends on various factors like the clinical details provided, expertise of the bioinformatician, availability of population specific variant databases, etc. These tests are difficult to perform and interpret in prenatal settings, when phenotype information is incomplete or evolving. False negative results or variants of uncertain significance or apparently unrelated variants are often found on these tests, complicating counseling and management. Hence, these tests should always be accompanied by pre and post-test counseling. In view of the complexity of these tests, such counseling should preferably be provided by a professional well versed with these technologies and their implications as relevant to prenatal settings. These professionals may be a clinical geneticist or a fetal medicine specialist with knowledge of genetics. Pretest counseling is important to apprise families of important aspects relevant for them for decision making process. These aspects include understanding how likely is the diagnosis of a genetic syndrome (diagnostic yield of the test), what are the likely outcome in postnatal period if the baby is affected with a genetic syndrome (prognosis of a genetic syndrome), how long test results will take and cost implications, and risks to the pregnancy with an invasive fetal sampling. In addition, as these tests may reveal some variants of uncertain clinical significance which may complicate decision making for the families, this should be informed to the families. The post-test counseling would depend on the test results. In case a pathogenic or likely pathogenic variant matching the imaging findings is detected in the report, the implications of the same and postnatal prognosis needs to be communicated to the family. If a genetic report does not reveal any significant variant, family can be reassured provided comprehensive genetic testing as mentioned in answer to question number 4 above. Limitations of genetic tests and emerging genetic diseases not detectable using current technologies resulting in a small residual risk despite negative test report needs to be briefly mentioned. Genetic tests may reveal variants of uncertain significance (VOUS) and laboratories may choose to report these due to phenotypic match. No reproductive decisions should be taken on basis of such VOUS as these may or may not be of any clinical consequence. All such patients should be referred to a clinical geneticist.

Q9. When should consultation with a geneticist sought?

Draft recommendations: A clinical geneticist should be consulted if: (1) The family history or prenatal imaging findings are highly suggestive of a genetic syndrome, as these cases may need in-depth analysis to enable choice of the right test for the pregnancy as well as affected individuals in the family, if any. (2) If emerging genetic tests like exome sequencing are being planned as these involve complex counseling issues. (3) If CMA or ES report reveals a VOUS. (4) If CMA and ES reports are negative but suspicion of a genetic syndrome is high.

Summary of evidence: Analysis of the family pedigree or type/pattern of anomaly/ies detected on imaging may indicate a high probability of a genetic syndrome in some families. As genetic syndromes may arise due to wide array of genomic variations such as chromosomal abnormalities, microdeletions/microduplications and single gene disorders, different genetic test technologies are required to investigate the same. A clinical geneticist can ascertain differential diagnoses by evaluation of affected family members, analysis of family pedigree or recognition of pattern of prenatal imaging. Guidance regarding choice of suitable genetic test for the fetus and/or the affected family member can be provided by the geneticist in such families to enable timely and resource effective decision making. In cases where a CMA is normal and an ES test is planned on the fetal sample, it is preferable to obtain consultation from a clinical geneticist, as this technology's use in prenatal settings is associated with complex issues. In case a CMA or ES report has revealed a VOUS, a clinical geneticist opinion is essential to enable genotype-phenotype correlation and implications of the variant on the pregnancy, if any. A VOUS is a variant which on basis of available literature cannot be conclusively classified as pathogenic, i.e., causative of disease or benign, i.e., of no clinical relevance. Such variants should never be used to take irreversible decisions. In some cases, there is a high index of suspicion of a genetic syndrome, either due to a family history or due to the type or pattern on anomalies seen in the fetus; and the CMA and ES report is negative. Such cases also need a clinical geneticist referral to understand whether the tests performed were adequate for that case scenario, and any residual risk remains which needs additional workup using alternative/advanced technologies like whole genome sequencing, exon array or gene specific MLPA.

ACKNOWLEDGMENT

I would like to acknowledge Dr Ratna Puri for proof reading and valuable suggestions.

BIBLIOGRAPHY

1. Aggarwal S, Tandon A, Das Bhowmik A, et al. A dysmorphology based systematic approach toward perinatal genetic diagnosis in a fetal autopsy series. Fetal Pediatr Pathol. 2018;37(1):49-68.
2. Armour CM, Dougan SD, Brock JA, et al.; On-Behalf-Of the Canadian College of Medical Geneticists. Practice guideline: joint CCMG-SOGC recommendations for the use of chromosomal microarray analysis for prenatal diagnosis and assessment of fetal loss in Canada. J Med Genet. 2018;55(4):215-21.
3. Dugoff L, Norton ME, Kuller JA. The use of chromosomal microarray for prenatal diagnosis. Am J Obstet Gynecol. 2016;215(4):B2-9.
4. Gagnon A; GENETICS COMMITTEE. Evaluation of prenatally diagnosed structural congenital anomalies. J Obstet Gynaecol Can. 2009;31(9):875-81.
5. International Society for Prenatal Diagnosis; Society for Maternal and Fetal Medicine; Perinatal Quality Foundation. Joint Position Statement from the International Society for Prenatal Diagnosis (ISPD), the Society for Maternal Fetal Medicine (SMFM), and the Perinatal Quality Foundation (PQF) on the use of genome-wide sequencing for fetal diagnosis. Prenat Diagn. 2018;38(1):6-9.
6. Mellis R, Chandler N, Chitty LS. Next-generation sequencing and the impact on prenatal diagnosis. Expert Rev Mol Diagn. 2018;18(8):689-99.
7. Monaghan KG, Leach NT, Pekarek D, et al.; ACMG Professional Practice and Guidelines Committee. The use of fetal exome sequencing in prenatal diagnosis: a points to consider document of the American College of Medical Genetics and Genomics (ACMG). Genet Med. 2020;22(4):675-80.
8. Oneda B, Rauch A. Microarrays in prenatal diagnosis. Best Pract Res Clin Obstet Gynaecol. 2017;42:53-63.
9. Phadke SR, Gupta A. Comparison of prenatal ultrasound findings and autopsy findings in fetuses terminated after prenatal diagnosis of malformations: an experience of a clinical genetics center. J Clin Ultrasound. 2010;38(5): 244-9.
10. Practice Bulletin No. 162: Prenatal diagnostic testing for genetic disorders. Obstet Gynecol. 2016;127(5):e108-22.

8

CHAPTER

Fetal Autopsy and Placental Pathology

Prakash Gambhir

Q1. Why fetal autopsy is necessary to investigate a fetal loss?

Draft recommendations:

- It is important to investigate each fetal loss/terminated fetus for congenital anomalies/intrauterine demise (IUD)/stillbirth to determine the cause of the loss.
- Fetal autopsy will enable us to have the diagnostic information as well as chance to sample the fetal tissues.
- Determining the etiology will help in counseling, choosing correct reproductive option, prevention of recurrence in future pregnancy by preconception antenatal management/prenatal diagnosis.
- Alongside fetus the placenta can also be studied to determine the cause of fetal loss.
- Various studies have shown that fetal autopsy gives important additional information in significant number of cases.

Summary of evidence: Efficacy of fetal autopsy as a diagnostic tool has been reported by studies. Fetal autopsy not only confirms the prenatal ultrasonography findings but also can elicit significant findings that can have impact on final diagnosis. Such additional information is rendered in 22–70% proving value of fetal autopsy. Though diagnostic yield of fetal autopsy may vary according to indication, still the diagnosis is reached in over 40% of cases in most of the categories and near 70% in many. Similarly, examination of placenta gives important information in IUDs and FGRs (fetal growth restriction). It is important to note that while we can study parents in future also, fetus and placenta can be studied only when they are available to us before disposal. It is also the last opportunity to obtain fetal tissues for DNA and other studies.

Research gap: Additional contribution of the next generation sequencing and array techniques to diagnostic yield in fetal autopsies needs to be studied further. Also the systematic studies of placenta and cord as per international standards and its contribution in causing IUDs and FGRs can be planned. Etiology of FGR and IUDs is not established in a significant proportion of cases.

Q2. What is the essential documentation for a fetal autopsy?

Draft recommendations:

- Informed consent is required preferably from both parents.
- Information that should be discussed with the parents before the consent is regarding the benefits and limitations of fetal autopsy, the actual process of autopsy, how will be the organs and tissues be dealt with after autopsy, and fetus disposal after autopsy.
- Parents should be assured that fetus will be treated with dignity and respect.
- It is necessary to record the delivery of the fetus and as per the law and hospital delivery records and death certificate should accompany the consent.
- Doctor's referring letter and antenatal investigations should also be provided.

Summary of evidence: The couple is in the state of grief and shock. Information that is provided when consent is obtained will help the couple to make the decision regarding the option of autopsy as well as help them to adjust to the bereavement. Parents should be encouraged to ask questions. They should be explained about the process of autopsy and what value as a diagnostic work up it will have. They should also be explained regarding what will happen to organs and tissues and how the fetus and fetal organs will be disposed after autopsy. If the couple does not want full autopsy other options like limited autopsy, imaging with MRI if available, tissue sampling can be discussed. Further investigations cytogenetic, molecular on fetal tissues should be discussed with the couple.

Research gap: All couples may not opt for fetal autopsy. Number of autopsies performed when compared to the number of the fetal losses/terminations/IUDs is miniscule. The reasons for this scenario warrant a study.

Q3. What are the essential components of fetal autopsy?

Draft recommendations:

Essential components of fetal autopsy are:

1. Informed consent
2. Clinical photograph
3. Fetogram
4. Morphometry
5. External examination
6. Dissection
7. Histopathology
8. Relevant sampling
9. DNA studies
10. Documentation

Summary of evidence: Informed consent should be an essential part of fetal autopsy. Clinical photographs should be obtained from fetus, cord, and placenta. Fetal whole body, face, front on, and lateral view should be obtained. Fetus, hands, and back should also be photographed. Any abnormality, if present, should have more detailed photographs. Fetal X-ray should be performed in every case. At least one front on view should be obtained and preferably a lateral view should accompany that. External measurements such as head circumference, chest, and abdominal circumference should be measured. Length, crown rump length, and various arm segment length should also be recorded. Inner and outer canthal distance should be measured for telorism. Foot length is an important parameter regarding gestation. After grossing all organs should be weighed. Dissection should be performed and organs should have gross inspection weight and sectioning for histopathology.

Histopathology, cytogenetic, and molecular studies on fetal DNA should be performed. All the images, consents, and reports should be documented and stored.

Research gap: Normal fetal phenotypes at various gestations may be different.

Q4. What are the different dissection techniques for fetal autopsy?

Draft recommendations: Autopsies should be performed by trained perinatal or fetal pathologists.

Various techniques for fetal autopsy are:

1. Virchow's technique (each organ dissected individually)
2. Rokitansky technique (in situ examination with removal of notable organs)
3. Letulle's technique (en mass removal of all the viscera)
4. Ghon's technique (en bloc dissection of thoracic, abdominal organs)

Summary of evidence: The incisions available are either T or Y shaped incision. The techniques that can be used are as per the choice of the pathologist or the anomalies in the fetus. Brain can also be approached either by median posterior or by transverse posterior parietal scalp incision. Posterior approach can be employed if posterior fossa lesions are expected. Prior fixation and removal under water are advisable.

Q5. How does imaging help in fetal autopsy?

Draft recommendations:

Imaging that is easily available.

1. *Clinical photographs:* They help in documentation, dysmorphology diagnosis through syndrome identification
2. *X-rays:* They help in identifying skeletal abnormalities and skeletal dysplasia, further elucidation of birth defects, calcifications and other

abnormalities detecting the conditions, ossification patterns, and gestation estimation.

Imaging that may not be universally available:

1. CT imaging
2. MRI

Summary of evidence: Simple radiologic imaging is available at all centers. Unlike ultrasonographic imaging radiologic studies cannot be performed antenatally. X-rays are diagnostic in most of the skeletal dysplasia and give important phenotypes that need to be correlated with the data from NGS studies. It gives important information in fetuses which do not have skeletal dysplasia also. In one large series it was noted that radiological imaging had significant findings in 30% of fetuses. It changed the impression in 8.6% of autopsies and was diagnostic in 3.1%. MRI is not available at all centers but can be used for noninvasive fetal evaluation where consent for full autopsy is not available.

Research gap: Comparison studies between full autopsy and MRI are not widely available. Fetal MRI infrastructure and expertise available at few centers only.

Q6. What is role of histopathology in fetal autopsy?

Draft recommendations: Histopathology of tissues and organs is an essential component of fetal autopsy and it characterizes the changes seen in prenatal ultrasonography images further. Thus it helps to achieve the diagnosis in fetal autopsy.

Following blocks should be obtained:

1. Thymus
2. Heart
3. lungs
4. Liver
5. Pancreas
6. Spleen
7. Adrenal glands
8. Kidneys
9. Muscle and diaphragm
10. Stomach, small and large intestines
11. *Bone:* Rib including growth plate in stillbirth; long bone (including growth plate), vertebral body and skull mandatory for suspected skeletal dysplasia
12. *Brain:* If preservation allows include cerebral cortex and periventricular white matter Deep gray matter near caudate nucleus, cerebellum, and pons.

Summary of evidence: The normal weight of the organs and the histopathology depends on the gestation of the fetus. Histopathology of organs adds further diagnostic inputs to the prenatally detected ultrasonographic findings especially for organs such as, kidneys, liver, and lungs.

Q7. What is the role of placental histopathology in fetal autopsy and how should it be performed and reported?

Draft recommendations:

- Placenta and cord examination is an integral part of fetal autopsy
- It should be reported as per the international standards

Summary of evidence: Placenta is called the diary of pregnancy. Placental histopathologic evaluation not only gives information about placental insufficiency but also about intrauterine infections and storage disorders. Cord examination also gives information regarding the cord accidents and possible malperfusion. The sectioning and grading of lesions along with the terminologies used should preferably be as per the Amsterdam consensus.

Q8. Which laboratory investigations, molecular, cytogenetic, and others should be performed alongside fetal autopsy?

Draft recommendations:

- DNA isolation should be performed in each fetal autopsy case.
- Selection of molecular test depends on the suspected diagnosis.
- For suspected chromosomal etiology cytogenetic microarray is preferred over karyotyping.
- For suspected monogenic disorders if a specific diagnosis is under consideration Sanger sequencing can be employed. Otherwise whole exome sequencing can be used.
- For diagnosis of intrauterine infections TORCH PCR can be used or other molecular infectious diagnosis can be employed.

Q9. How are the fetal tissues sampled for these investigations?

Draft recommendations:

- For DNA studies/cytogenetic investigations fetal skin 1 cm × 1 cm with underlying tissue should be collected from untouched part of the body.
- For placental tissue, preferable site is near the cord insertion at the placental end.
- These collections should be made at the hospital immediately after the delivery.
- Tissue culture medium should be made available prior to the procedure.
- Other tissues that can be used for studies are cord blood, liver, or spleen.

Q10. What are the essential things to be observed at the hospital/center where delivery is taking place?

Draft recommendations:

- To obtain informed consent from the couple.
- Referral prescription with delivery details and suspected diagnosis.
- Pregnancy and conception details
- Investigation reports, ultrasonography marker, and others.
- To arrange for a proper container prior to the procedure.
- To collect tissues for DNA/cytogenetic studies immediately postdelivery before placing in formalin.
- To put fetus and placenta in 10% formalin post collection of tissue sample.

Q11. If consent for full autopsy is not possible how can a minimally invasive/noninvasive autopsy be performed?

Draft recommendations: If consent for full autopsy is not available from the parents following options can be offered.

- External examination of the body with X-rays, clinical photographs and tissue sampling.
- Dissection limited to one or two body cavities.
- Open or needle biopsy of specific internal organs (as per indication)
- Placental studies, especially in IUDs and FGRs
- If available, CT/MRI alone or with targeted biopsies

BIBLIOGRAPHY

1. Fallet-Bianco C, Bie ID, Désilete V, et al. No. 365-Fetal and Perinatal Autopsy in Prenatally Diagnosed Fetal Abnormalities with Normal Chromosome Analysis. J Obstet Gynaecol Can. 2018;40(10):1358-66.e5.
2. Khong TY, Mooney EE, Ariel I, et al. Sampling and Definitions of Placental Lesions: Amsterdam Placental Workshop Group Consensus Statement. Arch Pathol Lab Med. 2016;140(7):698-713.
3. Puri RD, Kotecha U, Lall M, et al. Is the diagnostic yield influenced by the indication for fetal autopsy? Am J Med Genet A. 2016;170(8):2119-26.
4. Royal college of Pathologists. (2024). Guidelines on Autopsy practice. [online] Available from https://www.rcpath.org/static/1ebdc7d0-e84a-4fa4-895db816275a4391/82dbccb1-2285-42e0-907fc1d5e0719829/G193-Fetal-autopsy-associated-with-congenital-anomaly.pdf. [Last accessed November, 2024].
5. Thayyil S, Chitty LS, Robertson NJ, et al. Minimally invasive fetal postmortem examination using magnetic resonance imaging and computerised tomography: current evidence and practical issues. Prenat Diagn. 2010;30:713-8.
6. Varli IH, Petersson K, Botting R, et al. The Stockholm classification of stillbirth. Acta Obstet Gynecol Scand. 2008;87:1202-12.
7. Wainright HC. My approach to performing a perinatal or neonatal autopsy. J Clin Pathol. 2006;59:673-80.

CHAPTER 9

Approach to Intellectual Disability and/or Dysmorphism for Prenatal Diagnosis

Chaitanya A Datar

Q1. Why is there a need for a genetic consultation and diagnosis in an index child with ID ± dysmorphism for discussing recurrence risks and offering prenatal diagnosis in a pregnancy?

Draft recommendations:

- Genetic diagnosis in the index child or family with ID/dysmorphism is necessary to be able to discuss exact recurrence risks and offer prenatal diagnosis.
- Consultation with a geneticist is recommended to understand the inheritance patterns and significance of the variant in causing the disease state in the index case and/determine significance of variants identified on couple carrier screening.
- Understanding the risks will help the couple take informed decisions regarding prenatal diagnosis and the plan tests to be considered in the fetus.

Evidence: Global developmental delay and intellectual disability are phenotypically and genetically heterogeneous. A systematic clinical approach can help to identify a genetic cause for global developmental delay (GDD) and ID. Clinical geneticists have an expertise in genetic diagnostics, management of genetic conditions, and counseling services. Pediatric/obstetric healthcare providers might choose to refer to a genetics provider in cases where a specific genetic condition is suspected, additional etiological work-up is indicated after nondiagnostic testing, or the provider is not equipped to facilitate discussion and ordering of specific testing. Following receipt of results, the healthcare providers could also refer to medical geneticists given that medical geneticists are well-poised to facilitate clinical correlation of genomic variants, evaluation of VUS, and management of patients with genetic diagnoses. A clinical geneticist will review the medical, developmental, and antenatal history, consider a physical, dysmorphological and neurologic exam, and review of three-generation family history.

Though technological advances now allow for a specific genetic diagnosis to be identified in a substantial portion of affected individuals, still there may be a failure to identify definitive etiologic diagnosis in some cases or the possibility of identifying variants of unknown significance, incidental/

secondary findings, or unexpected information about familial relationships. These aspects must be clarified in the pre and post-test counseling sessions.

One of the important reasons for making a specific diagnosis in a child who presents with GDD is to allow accurate counseling of parents about recurrence risks and options for prenatal diagnosis and preimplantation genetic diagnosis.

Furthermore, genetic testing allows healthcare providers to refine recurrence risk counseling for the family to inform reproductive decision making. When an etiology is determined, the risk of recurrence for an individual family varies depending on the specific genomic variant(s) identified. This refined recurrence risk information offers patients, parents, and family members an understanding of their reproductive risks and informs reproductive decision making, restores reproductive confidence, and enables prenatal diagnosis. In the absence of an identifiable genetic etiology, empiric recurrence risk estimates are used.

Generally, recommendations stated that uncertainties should be addressed during pre- or post-test counseling. Also, pre- and post-test counseling should enable parents to make informed decisions about which results they wish to receive. Only two papers offered more specific direction on which points should always be discussed in pre- and/or post-test counseling and in which format(s) (e.g., written and orally). Several papers agreed counseling should be provided by a specialized genetic professional.

Gaps in literature: There are no studies to measure the outcomes of the impact of counseling for prenatal diagnosis and management. Some available studies qualitative studies are from the pre- or early genomic era. Post the advent of NGS (WES/WGS), genetic counseling has become more complex in the prenatal scenario and more formal studies in this domain are required.

Q2. When should the index child with ID ± dysmorphism ideally be tested for offering prenatal counseling and diagnosis?

Draft recommendations:

- Ideally all index cases with ID/dysmorphism must be tested for etiology and couple should be tested for carrier status before they plan a conception (preconceptional period).
- However, if the index child/couple miss the preconceptional evaluation, they must be referred to a clinical geneticist as soon as pregnancy is confirmed or at the first antenatal visit for testing and counseling.

Evidence: Prenatal diagnosis for major genetic disorders and congenital disabilities with a poor prognosis and discontinuation of the pregnancy, if the fetus is affected, is an accepted strategy for reducing the burden of genetic disorders. However, information about the correct test, appropriate time for ordering the test and expertise for pre-test and post-test counseling is often lacking.

In the context of beta thalassemia, Phadke et al. have mentioned that the best time to screen couples for thalassemia and hemoglobinopathies is prepregnancy or at the first antenatal visit preferably in the first trimester. This is the time when the couple/families are keenly interested in the well-being of the to-be-born child, more receptive to the information provided and are willing for immediate and appropriate actions. Over-enthusiastic groups have been advising premarital screening especially to screen for thalassemia carriers. Such actions affecting social behavior, usually do not have general acceptance by the population and may also stigmatize individuals causing problems with marriage proposals. Hence, this strategy is not advocated. Though discussed largely in the context of beta thalassemia, similar suggestions may be considered for other single gene conditions which often present as dysmorphism/ID.

Getting tested before pregnancy gives the couple a greater range of options and more time to make decisions and hence testing in index cases and parental carrier screening and counseling ideally should be performed before pregnancy.

Some researchers have noted that the best time to offer expanded carrier screening is during preconception or early in the first trimester to increase the likelihood of uptake. Preconception testing has the potential to identify whether partners are carriers of one of many known genetic disorders that could be passed to their fetus, and subsequent prenatal testing can identify if a fetus carries a genetic diagnosis. In some cases, preimplantation genetic diagnosis and embryo selection can be carried out, typically following genetic counseling, if the couple has resources and a desire to select for implantation of an unaffected embryo.

Genetic testing is time consuming and there must be sufficient time to test index child and parents. Also there may be significant anxiety if variants of uncertain significance are identified, and to take decisions regarding testing for these variants in an ongoing pregnancy may be stressful. Couple may occasionally have to consider concurrent testing in index child, themselves and the fetus which may cause a significant financial burden as well. Hence it is ideal to test index cases in the preconceptional period.

Gaps in literature: No definitive guidelines or studies have been formulated to discuss and suggest the timelines for performing testing in index cases and offering prenatal testing. Since index children are mostly following with pediatricians/relevant field specialists and the pregnancy is managed by an obstetrician, there is no common interface where both these issues are addressed together. Review of cases by clinical geneticist would perhaps offer that much needed cohesion between the two practitioners and thus aid in appropriate prenatal testing.

3. What are the indications of doing a karyotype, microarray and whole exome sequencing in cases where the index child has ID ± dysmorphism? What is the yield of each test in such cases?

Draft recommendations:

- G-banded karyotype analysis should be reserved for patients with obvious chromosomal syndromes (e.g., Down syndrome), a family history of chromosomal rearrangement, or a history of multiple miscarriages only.
- Use of CMA in place of standard karyotyping as the first-tier cytogenetic diagnostic test in the clinical evaluation of children with DD/ID/ASDs, especially when associated with dysmorphic features and/cardiac anomalies.
- Whole exome sequencing may be preferred over disease based panels for next-generation sequence-based tests. However, a proper phenotyping by a clinical geneticist or a trained Clinician is necessary before ordering this test.
- WES has a higher yield in cases with neurological symptoms associated with ID/dysmorphism.

Evidence: Submicroscopic chromosomal rearrangements are the most common identifiable causes of intellectual disability and autism spectrum disorders associated with dysmorphic features. Chromosomal microarray (CMA) can detect copy number variants <1 Mb. Battaglia et al. studied 349 individuals with the above features, and 91 CNVs were detected in 77 patients with a high yield of 22.06%. Of these cases, 5 (6.49%) presented with borderline cognitive impairment, 54 (70.13%) with a variable degree of DD/ID, and 18/77 (23.38%) with ID of variable degree and ASD. The CNVs caused the phenotype in 57/77 (74%) patients; 12/57 (21.05%) had ASDs/ID, and 45/57 (78.95%) had DD/ID. This study provides evidence of the high diagnostic yield of CMA for genetic testing in children with unexplained ID/ASDs who had dysmorphic features.

CMA offers a much higher diagnostic yield (15%–20%) for genetic testing of individuals with unexplained DD/ID, ASD, or MCA than a G-banded karyotype (~3%, excluding Down syndrome and other recognizable chromosomal syndromes), essentially because of its higher sensitivity for submicroscopic deletions and duplications. Truly balanced rearrangements and low-level mosaicism are generally not detectable by arrays, but these are relatively infrequent causes of abnormal phenotypes in the population (<1%). Available evidence strongly supports the use of CMA in place of G-banded karyotyping as the first-tier cytogenetic diagnostic test for patients with DD/ID, ASD, or MCA. G-banded karyotype analysis should be reserved for patients with obvious chromosomal syndromes (e.g., Down syndrome), a family history of chromosomal rearrangement, or a history of multiple miscarriages.

Two forms of CMA that are implemented in the genomic analysis; these being, array comparative genomic hybridization (aCGH) and single nucleotide polymorphism (SNP) array. In comparison to aCGH, microarray-based SNP analysis has the potential to detect instances of uniparental disomy (UPD) and lower grade mosaicism (~5%).

Fluorescent in situ hybridization (FISH) testing is limited to cases in which the patient's phenotype is indicative of a definite disorder such that the precise probe can be utilized. Therefore, it may be utilized for the identification of syndromes associated with DD/ID such as Angelman syndrome, Prader–Willi syndrome, and velocardiofacial/DiGeorge syndrome (VCFS/DGS), William syndrome etc.

Whole exome sequencing (WES) can be utilized to identify a causative genomic variant in an individual presenting with DD/ID with associated dysmorphic features for whom conventional testing such as CMA was unrevealing.

The patients with multiple congenital anomalies might have a higher detection rate of CNVs than other ID patients. Therefore, the ID patients may be subdivided into 3 subgroups, including ID with MCA, ID with ASD and other IDs. The diagnostic yield and variation types were different in different ID subgroups. ID with MCA subgroup showed a higher detection rate of CNVs. ID with ASD showed the lowest detection rate in both CNVs and SNVs. More single-nucleotide variations were identified in other ID subgroups.

In a study of a large cohort of 100 patients, Wang et al studied the clinical characteristics of patients, with congenital anomalies or dysmorphic features, and these seemed mostly unrelated to the WES outcome, while presence of unexplained epilepsy and ID seemed to show a higher yield. Another study retrospectively analyzed 48 subjects (18 females, 30 males; median age: 7.5 years) using single gene panels. It is expected that up to 40% patients with ID could likely have a monogenic form. Consanguinity was present in 17%, autism in 38%, seizures in 42%, nonspecific dysmorphic features in 67%, and abnormalities on neurological examination in 56%. The diagnostic yield was 21% (10/48) overall, and 38% with the more recent trio-based panel.

The advantage of using whole exome panels over targeted disease based panels is highlighted by the fact that some genes could exclusively cause a particular phenotype and hence may be absent in other gene panels and also the possibility of a blended phenotype where 2 different genes are causative of the clinical presentation. It may be expensive and cumbersome to use separate panels, hence whole exome sequencing can be the test of choice especially where the phenotype is unclear or mixed.

Snoeijen-Schouwenaars et al. observed that full exome analysis also has the advantage of the possible identification of novel or very recently discovered new genes for phenotypes with both ID and epilepsy that have not yet been included in current panel releases. In addition, full exome analysis allows a genome-wide analysis for chromosomal copy number variations and can thereby largely replace separate chromosomal analysis by array analysis.

Notably, there is emerging evidence based on two recent meta-analyses that ES and possibly GS should be considered as a first-tier test for the diagnostic evaluation of individuals with NDDs. Clark et al. (2018) conducted a meta-analysis of 37 studies encompassing 20,068 children with a range of indications including NDDs and found that the diagnostic yields of GS (41%) and ES (36%) were substantially greater than CMA (10%) in these children with suspected genetic diseases. Furthermore, in this meta-analysis, the clinical utility, defined as change in clinical management, of GS (27%) and ES (17%) were higher than of CMA (6%). Srivastava et al. (2019) conducted a meta-analysis of ES in patients with isolated NDDs and NDDs plus associated conditions (e.g., syndromic features, systemic findings, and neurologic features). Based on 30 studies comprising 3,350 patients, the diagnostic yield of ES (31% in isolated NDD, 53% in NDD plus associated conditions, and 36% overall) was substantially higher than the generally accepted diagnostic yield of CMA (10%–20%).

Gaps in literature: There is evidence still emerging about the utility of WES in cases with ID/dysmorphism. New syndromic diagnosis and identification of variants of uncertain significance coupled with inadequate phenotyping or variability of phenotypic presentations are complicating the picture. The advent of whole genome sequencing could pave way for evaluation of larger copy number variants being analyzed and thus making CMA a redundant test. But more studies will be needed and literature needs to keep up with the rapid pace at which genomic technology is progressing and evolving.

Q4. Is it ideal to consider whole exome sequencing in the index child with ID ± dysmorphism alone (single) or as a trio with parents?

Draft recommendations:

- Solo exome sequencing may be more cost effective approach if the phenotype is well defined.
- There is a better diagnostic yield of trio exome sequencing (index case and parents together) in cases of Intellectual disability where the clinical spectrum can be non-specific and, with sometimes complicated due to incomplete penetrance and variable expressivity.

- There is a higher possibility of identifying de novo mutations pertaining to dominant genes especially in non-consanguineous families with simplex cases. In these cases trio testing has a better diagnostic yield.
- Trio testing helps in a better resolution of variants of uncertain significance identified in relation to the ID phenotype and aids in a faster diagnosis especially when prenatal testing needs to be considered for the couple's ongoing pregnancy.

Evidence: Myriam Srour et al. retrospectively analyzed 48 subjects (median age: 7.5 years) using next-generation sequencing panels for ID genes. The diagnostic yield was 21% (10/48) overall, and 38% with the more recent trio-based panel. Eight of 10 patients had *de novo* pathogenic dominant mutations, one had an inherited pathogenic autosomal dominant mutation, and one had compound heterozygous pathogenic recessive mutations. Consanguinity was present in 17% of these cases. Intellectual disability could be caused by *de novo* variants in approximately 45–55% of patients after exclusion of copy number variations. Trio-based exome sequencing is helpful in identifying *de novo* alterations and pathologic genes, if all patients undergo trio-based exome analysis, the yield of diagnosis would increase.

Mau-Them et al. 2019, observed that in cases with developmental disorders, a second step trio-based exome sequencing analysis appears an efficient strategy to improve the diagnostic yield and trio-ES strategy increased the initial diagnostic yield of solo-ES from about 30%–49% in the selected cohort where trio testing was performed. They propose a solo-ES for patient with specific phenotypic description and suspected Mendelian disorders and trio-ES for all other patients. But, in the DD/ID cases, patients often present with a clinical spectrum of nonspecific symptoms, with sometimes incomplete penetrance and variable expressivity. However, in cost limited situations considering solo-ES as first-tier strategy for every patient followed by a trio-ES in the negative patients yet appears more efficient.

Solo-ES is time consuming because of the numerous missense variants and the enrichment of missense among the VOUS. But, trio-ES's main disadvantage is the cost generated from additional parental ES. Nevertheless, this cost is expected to decrease and can also be counterbalanced since trio-ES drastically reduces the biological (variant interpretation) and technical (Sanger validation) costs, especially regarding interpretation of missense variants.

Numerous studies have found a high diagnostic yield of ES—potentially >40% in patients with ID and other NDDs, especially when performed as a trio including both biological parents. Alfares et al. observed that in their majorly consanguineous cohort, there was no significant difference between solo versus trio testing. But the trio-based analysis was a better approach and each additional family member helped to narrow down the number of variants by 50–75%. The other advantage of trio testing was reducing the turnaround time and providing results faster than by performing segregation analysis for the candidate variants. While solo exome testing might provide the best clinical practice in our population, there might be other scenarios in which extended analysis is required, such as when results are urgently required for an ongoing pregnancy, when other family members might not be available in future visits or when segregation analysis for any identified variant is not possible.

Gaps in literature: More studies are required to study advantages of solo versus trio exome pertaining to the yield and cost effectiveness. The Indian population needs to be reviewed specifically in the context of significant consanguinity and endogamy.

Q5. Is Fragile X testing necessary for all male/female index cases with ID and which is the test of choice?

Draft recommendations:

- Fragile X syndrome testing must be considered in all males and females with global developmental delay/intellectual disability/autism of unknown cause.
- All individuals older than 50 years with ataxia and tremors or females with premature ovarian insufficiency or mild emotional/learning problems should be tested for this premutation. Family history for these conditions must be inquired in all cases where the proband presents with ID.
- Testing should be done by triplet primed PCR and followed up with Southern blot testing if necessary.

Evidence: Fragile X syndrome (FXS) is the most prevalent inherited cause of mild-to-severe intellectual disability and the most common monogenic cause of autism spectrum disorder. It accounts for about one-half of cases of X-linked intellectual disability and is the most common cause of mental impairment after trisomy 21. Triplet repeat expansion mutations (CGG repeats) in *FMR1* gene cause Fragile X syndrome. CGG repeats: Normal—5–44 repeats, intermediate—45–54 repeats, premutation—55–200, full mutation (with methylation) > 200 repeats.

Fragile X testing should be performed in all boys and girls with GDD/ID/autism of unknown cause. In boys with GDD/ID/autism of uncertain cause, 2–3% will have Fragile X syndrome (full mutation of *FMR1*, >200 CGG repeats), as will 1–2% of girls (full mutation). In addition, all individuals older than 50 years with ataxia and tremors or females with premature ovarian insufficiency, mild emotional/learning problems should be tested for this premutation. Family history for the above signs/symptoms must be inquired in at least three generations. Testing is not routinely warranted in cases with isolated attention deficit hyperactivity disorder.

Diagnosis of Fragile X syndrome must be confirmed through molecular testing by double-or triple-primer PCR plus capillary electrophoresis, which quantifies the number of triplets. The diagnosis must be confirmed by Southern blot, which provides the activation ratio of the X chromosome in women with Fragile X syndrome and detects copy number mosaicism in men and women. When these tests are negative, but the clinical suspicion of Fragile X syndrome persists, WES, and WGS are suggested. Cytogenetic studies, i.e., karyotyping and microarray should not be used for testing for Fragile X syndrome.

Gaps in literature: Males with mild ID/ASD and females with mild ID/ASD or learning disabilities are not tested for FXS, hence the exact incidence could be underestimated. Frequency of point variations in the FXS promoter region which could cause FXS in TP-PCR negative cases needs to be studied. WGS is expected to diagnose FXS, but evidence in this regard must be generated before shifting to the newer technology for an accurate diagnosis.

Q6. Is prenatal diagnosis for an ongoing pregnancy indicated for a variant of uncertain significance (VOUS) identified in an index child with ID ± dysmorphism on whole exome sequencing or microarray?

Draft recommendations:

- Variants of uncertain significance (VOUS) in index cases with ID/ dysmorphism may be considered for prenatal testing if there is a good genotype-phenotype correlation and parental segregation has been carried out.
- It is recommended to have the case reviewed by a clinical geneticist or a specialist trained in Genetics before considering VOUS variants for prenatal testing.
- Periodic reanalysis of data and reclassification of VOUS variants must be considered, especially before offering prenatal diagnosis under the guidance of a clinical geneticist or a relevant specialist.

Evidence: Exome sequencing (ES) has enhanced the diagnostic yield of genetic testing in cases with ID and dysmorphism, but has also increased the possibility of uncertain findings. Laboratory specialists are challenged to interpret results. Clinicians are challenged to return results that have an element of uncertainty in a way that is understandable to parents. Parents are challenged to apply meaning to this information, and decide about the course of their pregnancy based on results that may not provide the certainty that they had hoped for.

In a cohort including ID cases, pathogenic or likely pathogenic variants were found in 100 individuals (27%), with variants of uncertain significance in an additional 42 (11.3%). Through systematic reanalyzes, the authors could reclassify 15 variants, with 11.3% of families who initially were found to harbor a VUS and 4.7% of families with a negative result eventually found to harbor a pathogenic or likely pathogenic variant.

The authors have demonstrated the value of systematic reanalysis, which has thus far yielded Pathogenic/Likely Pathogenic variants for an additional 17 individuals (17% of total P/LP variation, 4.6% of total probands). Given the rates of progress in Mendelian disease genetics and the development of new genomic annotations, they believe that systematic reanalysis of genomic data should become standard practice.

In order to protect pregnant couples from the burden of uncertain results, the genetic professionals have to take the responsibility to limit the reporting of VUS. However, some authors stated that reporting VUS matching the phenotype may be considered (Lazier et al., 2022; Monaghan et al., 2020).

Matthijs et al. (2016) stated that in a diagnostic ES setting, analysis should only include genes with established phenotype-genotype correlations. According to Richards et al. (2015) VUS sequence variants should not be used in clinical decision making, however, Dugoff et al. (2016) suggested reporting VUS, but only after extensive pre- and post-test counseling.

It is extensively recommended to discuss the possibility of finding a VUS with the prospective couple during pretest counseling. Reporting a VUS, requires extensive post-test counseling by a clinical geneticist. It has been advised that when VUS are reported, it should be communicated to the prospective parent(s) that prenatal centers may have different policies (Monaghan et al., 2020).

Pre- and post-test counseling were considered important in guiding patients through uncertainty. During pre-test counseling, a genetic healthcare professional should obtain clinical information and consent. The types of variants that will be reported should be included in the consent document.

It may be advised to consider a trio analysis to aid interpretation and decision-making concerning reporting, by improving variant classification, discovering de novo variants or compound heterozygosity efficiently, or formally confirming a diagnosis.

Careful classification of variants is crucial for correct reporting. However, it was recommended to issue a new report to the clinician when categorization of a variant changes significantly, for example from (likely) pathogenic to (likely) benign. This possibility should be communicated with parents during post-test counseling. Other reanalyzes can be requested by the patient through their clinician, especially in case of a future pregnancy, after considerable time (e.g., >12 months), if the ES report did not comprise a complete phenotype, or the phenotype has expanded postnatally.

Local decision-making was highlighted as an important factor in handling uncertainty. The decision to report problematic variants (VUS, IF's, SF's, etc.) for example, often depends on multidisciplinary team and/or policies that are put in place either by a country or laboratory.

Gaps in literature: There are no clear guidelines in literature that advice regarding the inclusion of VOUS for prenatal testing. It is difficult to have common consensus guidelines in this regard as there are many confounding factors including-quality of phenotyping in index case, quality of the laboratory where the data is being handled, variant segregation in the family, etc. Most of the variant classification relies on Western data, which is found to have significant differences compared to our Indian population data. Generation of local population and lab databases and unification of these systems throughout the country will be required to handle VOUSes. More studies are necessary to be able to generate clear guidelines, but ambiguity is likely to remain since these variants are highly case based and individual clinicians will need to take a stand in this regard.

Q7. What if a patient presents with an advanced pregnancy and has an index child with ID ± dysmorphism who is yet undiagnosed? Can concurrent testing on index case, parents and fetus be performed to obtain a result within a limited time frame?

Draft recommendations:

- Solo testing of fetus by exome sequencing for an undiagnosed ID/ dysmorphism in the index child is not recommended.
- If the index child is undiagnosed and the gestational age is advanced, trio testing in proband and parents and concurrent fetal testing can be considered (quad testing).
- It is recommended to consider proper pre- and post-test counseling with a clinical geneticist or a specialist trained in Genetics before and after considering concurrent testing.

Evidence: For ES, trio/quad analysis is recommended to aid clinical interpretation. Diderich et al. observed that the process of variant classification in a prenatal setting faces several limitations: Incomplete fetal phenotype, insufficient (in silico) information to classify some variants as (likely) pathogenic or (likely) benign and no or partial knowledge on prenatal presentations of known syndromes. These limitations form a special challenge, also due to the limited time for executing the experiment and reporting the results (Lewis et al., 2021).

Trio-based study design allows rapid identification of de novo variants, which are enriched among variants that are causally related to deleterious pediatric phenotypes. However, in these cases incomplete penetrance requires caution as a parent carrying a certain variant may not be affected, while the variant may be(come) penetrant in the fetus. It is evident that most P/LP variants can be found within probands analyzed without parental information; however, additional curation time would be required in certain cases. In contrast to P/LP variants, VUSs would have been more difficult to identify without parental sequencing, owing to the fact that many VUSs do not affect genes known to associate with disease. Also, those VUSs that do affect genes known to associate with disease tended to have lower CADD ranks.

It is generally advised to consider trio analysis to aid interpretation and decision-making concerning reporting, by improving variant classification, discovering de novo variants or confirming the compound heterozygosity efficiently, and thus formally confirming a diagnosis. With regards to the laboratory report, determination of cis or trans of variants, or identification of multiple pathogenic variants, may be more effective with trio/quad analysis.

Trio analysis is recommended to improve diagnostic yield and obtain results faster, which is especially important in the prenatal context. Also trio-based sequencing is more sensitive and analytically efficient than proband-only sequencing. Further, VUSs and novel candidates are more difficult to identify without parental sequence data.

However, the importance of local policy and protocols, discussion of findings in multidisciplinary teams and proper pre- and post-test counseling is emphasized before any action on the trio result with concurrent fetal testing.

Gaps in literature: Data of concurrent testing in index, parents and fetus is limited in the general literature and has not been adequately evaluated in the Indian context. The Indian genomic scenario is unique in view of population differences from the Western data and high incidence of consanguinity and endogamy. The challenges of resolving VOUS in these cases is therefore more difficult. There are no uniform country-wide or laboratory policies that would guide variant interpretation, classification and reporting.

Q8. How to counsel families where genetic test has not yielded a significant/pathogenic variant? What is the residual risk of recurrence that must be discussed?

Draft recommendations:

- In cases where the index case is undiagnosed or testing has not yielded any significant P/LP variants or significant VUS, it is necessary to discuss empiric residual risks.
- This risk estimation must be given after searching the latest literature pertaining to the related disorder or phenotype. Genetic counseling by a clinical geneticist is recommended in such cases.

Evidence: At-risk families are mostly identified after the birth of an affected child or an informative family history and offered appropriate genetic counseling with the option of prenatal diagnosis for the condition under consideration.

In the absence of an identifiable genetic etiology, empiric recurrence risk estimates are used. There are several limitations in using empiric recurrence risks for NDDs. Over time, diagnostic criteria for certain NDDs change and study populations may be limited in size, compromising the accuracy of the risk estimates. In the 2013 ACMG guidelines, Schaefer et al. 2013, stated that the accepted recurrence risk for full siblings of a child with ASD is in the range of 3–10%. As reviewed by Schaefer (2016), it is now recommended to provide a 10–20% recurrence risk for full siblings of a child with ASD and a 30–50% risk if there is more than one affected sibling. Empiric recurrence risk for a full sibling of a child with ID is ~3% and increases to 10% if a parent is also diagnosed with ID (Harper 2010). Genetic counselors have an especially important role in helping parents make informed family planning decisions and cope with the fear of recurrence when there is not a single definitive probability of recurrence.

Gaps in literature: Estimation of residual risks for each condition if difficult since each of them is clinically heterogeneous. Literature in this regard is sparse and likely to change over time as more evidence would build up.

BIBLIOGRAPHY

1. Acero-Garcés DO, Saldarriaga W, Cabal-Herrera AM, et al. Fragile X Syndrome in children. Colomb Med (Cali). 2023;54(2):e4005089.
2. Alfares A, Alsubaie L, Aloraini T, et al. What is the right sequencing approach? Solo VS extended family analysis in consanguineous populations. BMC Med Genomics. 2020;13(1):103.
3. Bowling KM, Thompson ML, Amaral MD, et al. Genomic diagnosis for children with intellectual disability and/or developmental delay. Genome Med. 2017; 9:43.
4. Committee Opinion No. 691: Carrier Screening for Genetic Conditions. Obstet Gynecol. 2017;129(3):e41-55.
5. Diderich KEM, Klapwijk JE, van der Schoot V, et al. The role of a multidisciplinary team in managing variants of uncertain clinical significance in prenatal genetic diagnosis. Eur J Med Genet. 2023;66(10):104844.
6. Genetic Counseling in Neurodevelopmental Disorders. Cold Spring Harb Perspect Med. 2020;10(4):a036533.
7. Jo YH, Choi SH, Yoo HW, et al. Clinical use of whole exome sequencing in children with developmental delay/intellectual disability. Pediatr Neonatol. 2024;65(5):445-50.
8. Klapwijk JE, Srebniak MI, Go ATJI, et al. How to deal with uncertainty in prenatal genomics: a systematic review of guidelines and policies. Clin Genet. 2021;100(6):647-58.

9. Miller DT, Adam MP, Aradhya S, et al. Consensus statement: chromosomal microarray is a first-tier clinical diagnostic test for individuals with developmental disabilities or congenital anomalies. Am J Hum Genet. 2010;86(5):749-64.
10. Moeschler JB, Shevell M; Committee on Genetics. Comprehensive Evaluation of the Child With Intellectual Disability or Global Developmental Delays. Pediatrics. 2014;134(3):e903-18.
11. Parisi MA, Caggana M, Cohen JL. When is the best time to screen and evaluate for treatable genetic disorders?: a lifespan perspective. Am J Med Genet C Semin Med Genet. 2023;193(1):44-55.
12. Pekeles H, Accogli A, Boudrahem-Addour N, et al. Diagnostic yield of intellectual disability gene panels. Pediatr Neurol. 2019;92:32-6.
13. Phadke SR, Puri RD, Ranganath P. Prenatal screening for genetic disorders: suggested guidelines for the Indian Scenario. Indian J Med Res. 2017;146(6): 689-99.
14. Savatt JM, Myers SM. Genetic testing in neurodevelopmental disorders. Front Pediatr. 2021;9:526779.
15. Snoeijen-Schouwenaars FM, van Ool JS, Verhoeven JS, et al. Diagnostic exome sequencing in 100 consecutive patients with both epilepsy and intellectual disability. Epilepsia. 2019;60:155-64.
16. Tan TY, Lunke S, Chong B, et al. A head-to-head evaluation of the diagnostic efficacy and costs of trio versus singleton exome sequencing analysis. Eur J Hum Genet. 2019;27(12):1791-9.

CHAPTER 10

Genetic of Recurrent Pregnancy Loss

Hema Purandarey

Q1. What is the definition and main causes of RPL?

Draft recommendations: A diagnosis of recurrent pregnancy loss (RPL) could be considered if there are two or more documented 1st trimester pregnancy losses or one 2nd trimester loss including IVF pregnancies by ultrasound or histopathology of the tissue from previous marriages or current marriage.

Main causes of RPL can be subdivided into:
- Cytogenetic causes
- Hereditary and acquired thrombophilia including antiphospholipid syndrome
- Autoimmune disorders
- Anatomical
- Endocrine or metabolic causes
- Infections
- Male factors
- Psychological
- Alloimmune
- Other environmental, occupational, or personal habits

Summary of evidence: Recurrent pregnancy loss is a complex health challenge with no universally accepted definition. Due to the heterogeneity of definitions and criteria applied by international guidelines for recurrent pregnancy loss, the true incidence of recurrent miscarriage, which is reported to range from 1% to 5%, is difficult to estimate.

ESHRE 2022 recommends the above-mentioned definition for RPL.

RCOG green top guideline 2023 defines recurrent miscarriage as three or more miscarriages, while **ASRM 2012** says that for epidemiological purposes RPL should be defined as three or more consecutive losses, while, clinical evaluation may be initiated following two first trimester losses.

Evidence gap: Majority of recurrent pregnancy losses (50%) still remain unexplained and research is needed to explore the potential causes in these cases.

Q2. When should the cytogenetic factors be investigated?

Draft recommendations:

- Cytogenetic analysis should be offered on products of conception of the second or third and subsequent miscarriage(s) and in any second trimester miscarriage. An earlier evaluation is considered in cases of advanced maternal age or known genetic risk factors in the family history.
- The incidence of aneuploidy in recurrent miscarriage is found to be approximately 40%. Microarray techniques report even higher number of cytogenetic anomalies in women with sporadic miscarriages of up to 59.4%. Chromosomal microarray (CMA) on products of conception at the time of the second pregnancy loss will provide an explanation in more than 90% of cases. Finding of an aneuploid embryo has been found to confer an improved prognosis in the subsequent pregnancy.
- Analysis by conventional karyotyping is limited by the failure of tissue culture in 50% of cases and does not distinguish between maternal contamination and a normal (euploid) female fetus.
- Parental peripheral blood karyotyping should be offered for couples in whom POC testing has reported an unbalanced structural chromosomal abnormality or there is unsuccessful or no pregnancy tissue available for testing.

Summary of evidence:

ESHRE 2022 recommends that genetic analysis of pregnancy tissue following pregnancy loss has the benefit of providing the patient with a reason for the pregnancy loss and may help to determine whether further investigations or treatments are required.

CMA as the preferred modality for genetic testing in miscarriages as it is not limited by tissue culture failure or false-negative results secondary to maternal cell contamination and will reveal aneuploidy in about 55% of cases.

RCOG green top guideline 2023 recommends cytogenetic analysis should be offered on pregnancy tissue of the third and subsequent miscarriage(s) and in any second trimester miscarriage.

Evidence gap: Cost benefit analysis for the routine use of cytogenetic analysis of products of conception (POCs) needs to be carried out for its widespread implementation in low-resource settings.

Q3. How important are pretest genetic counseling and history taking for the diagnosis and prognosis of RPL?

Draft recommendation: Pretest genetic counseling with detailed elucidation of sensitivity, specificity, and cost effectiveness of the advised test, and personal and three generations familial, medical, and reproductive history taking are vital in diagnosis and management of RPL as they facilitate a comprehensive assessment of risk factors, guide personalized diagnostic and therapeutic strategies, provide psychological support, and improve overall prognosis by enabling informed decision-making and proactive management.

Poor prognostic factors for a subsequent chance of live birth include:

- Greater number of previous pregnancy losses
- Advanced maternal age
- Advanced paternal age
- Women with BMI <19 kg/m^2 or >25 kg/m^2
- Maternal smoking
- Paternal smoking
- Primary RPL
- Excess alcohol consumption
- Excess caffeine consumption
- Black ethnic background
- History of IVF/ICSI treatment—46% reduced odds

Summary of evidence:
ESHRE 2022 recommends the use of prognostic tools (such as those provided by Kolte and Westergaard) to provide an estimate of subsequent chance of live birth in couples with RPL.

ESHRE 2022 also states that most perilous time for women with idiopathic RPL was between 6 and 8 weeks of gestation. By 8 weeks of gestation, if a fetal heartbeat had been identified, the chances of a successful outcome in a subsequent pregnancy were 98%, climbing to 99.4% at 10 weeks of gestation.

Evidence gap: There are limited studies examining environmental chemical exposure and dietary intake; association, and the effects of these need to be further investigated.

Q4. What is the cytogenetic evaluation algorithm for products of conception (POC) with or without congenital abnormalities in singleton and multiple pregnancies?

Draft recommendations: For both singleton and multiple pregnancy losses, appropriate collection, preservation and transportation of tissue are critical for the success of cell growth in culture and the subsequent karyotype analysis. At receipt of the POC sample, the type and quality of tissue, mode of conception, and obstetric history with ultrasound reports (including chorionicity) are noted, with information about parental age, consanguinity, and ethnicity (though this is not reported to play a major role, it can refer to the potential risk of additional single gene disorders) and a thorough familial and personal obstetric and medical history with pertinent reports are collected and a pedigree chart is drawn accordingly.

Cytogenetic abnormalities in POCs can be detected by different techniques: Conventional G-band karyotyping, fluorescence in situ hybridization (FISH), multiplex ligation dependent probe amplification (MLPA), array comparative genomic hybridization (aCGH), single-nucleotide polymorphism (SNP) microarray and, recently, next-generation sequencing (NGS). Out of these array-CGH is recommended based on a reduced maternal contamination effect.

Summary of evidence:
ESHRE 2022 recommends array-CGH as the preferred method of genetic analysis, as this is not limited by tissue culture failure or false-negative results due to maternal cell contamination. However, array-CGH has some limitations with regard to not being able to detect balanced rearrangements and low-level mosaicism.

ASRM 2012 recognizes that there are pitfalls to this approach such as: The possibility of maternal tissue contamination of the specimen; failure to seek other causes of RPL if cytogenetic assessment reveals an abnormal karyotype; and the occurrence of noncytogenetic embryonic abnormalities.

Evidence gap: Role and benefit of newer techniques such as next-generation sequencing (NGS), whole genome screening (WGS), and whole exome screening (WES) needs to be explored.

Q5. How important are the male and female components of parental evaluation?

Draft recommendations: In cases of RPL, POC evaluated or unevaluated, the assessment starts with the current standard RPL evaluation.

Female components:
- Maternal testing for acquired thrombophilia, particularly for lupus anticoagulant, anticardiolipin antibodies, and β2 glycoprotein I antibodies.
- Women with second trimester miscarriage may be offered testing for Factor V Leiden, prothrombin gene mutation and protein C and S deficiency.
- Assessment for congenital uterine anomalies, ideally with 3D ultrasound.
- Thyroid function tests and assessment for thyroid peroxidase (TPO) antibodies.
- Pregestational diabetes
- *Lifestyle modifications:* Women with RPL should be advised to maintain a BMI between 19 kg/m^2 and 25 kg/m^2, smoking cessation, limit alcohol consumption and limit caffeine to less than 200 mg/day.

Male components: In male partner routine semen analysis is generally used to evaluate motility, count, and abnormal forms for fertility parameters.

Triploidy can result via dispermy, in which two sperm fertilize a single ovum. Mosaicism can result from aberrant postzygotic cell division. Additionally, in RPL cases, sperm DNA fragmentation is performed, and in severe cases of oligospermia, azoospermia, and teratozoospermia, the Y microdeletion test is carried out. It is known that spermatogenetic failure and male infertility are caused by Y chromosome microdeletion. Sperm aneuploidy screen by sperm FISH studies for five major chromosomes 13; 18; 21, X; and Y can be helpful in the assessment of male infertility and recurrent pregnancy loss.

Although there appears to be an association between sperm DNA fragmentation and miscarriage, there are yet to be any prospective trials demonstrating improved outcomes with intervention, hence, sperm DNA testing is not routinely recommended.

Parental karyotyping should be performed for couples in whom testing of pregnancy tissue reports an unbalanced structural chromosomal abnormality. It can also be offered when cytogenetic analysis is indicated but testing of the pregnancy tissue is unsuccessful or there is no pregnancy tissue available for testing.

Chromosomally normal parents can produce abnormal gametes by nondisjunction rearrangement or other mutational mechanisms such as crossing over errors, chromosomal breakage and misrepair and/or chromosomal instability.

Summary of evidence:
RCOG green top guideline 2023 recommends the aforementioned protocol.

ESHRE 2022 additionally recommends:

- Antinuclear antibodies (ANA) testing could be considered for explanatory purposes.
- All women with RPL should have 2D ultrasound to rule out adenomyosis.
- Assessing sperm DNA fragmentation in couples with RPL could be considered for diagnostic purposes.

Evidence gap: There is a growing body of evidence showing strong association between sperm DNA damage and RPL, however its implementation in in clinical settings to improve pregnancy outcomes needs more research.

Q6. What are the main effects of numerical and structural and chromosomal abnormalities, how do they occur and what needs to be done?

Draft recommendation: Approximately 50% of sporadic and 40% of recurrent miscarriages are a result of fetal chromosome anomalies. Among these are trisomy (51.9%); polyploidy (18.8%); monosomy (15.2%); structural anomalies (6.5%); and others (7.6%).

There are currently no clinically available options to repair genetic abnormalities. Thus, intervention is primarily based on preventative methods, either by using donor gametes or by embryo screening using preimplantation genetic diagnosis (PGD) to test for specific genetic abnormalities such as a known recessive genetic disorder and preimplantation genetic screening (PGS) to screen for copy number variations such as aneuploidy.

Summary of evidence: The mechanism of numerical chromosomal abnormality is nondisjunction at meiosis I or meiosis II. In meiosis I, homologous chromosomes fail to separate and migrate together to one cell. At meiosis II, sister chromatids fail to separate and migrate together to one cell. A higher rate of meiotic errors is typically linked to aberrant segregation during oocyte development in advanced maternal age.

The commonly known and observed abnormalities are monosomy, trisomy, polyploidy, mosaicism (including gonadal), structural abnormality (translocation, deletion, duplication caused by various breakages and rearrangements), Marker chromosome, X-linked recessive disorders, triple X pattern, and/or asymmetric inactivation of the X chromosome.

Aneuploidy: Presence of a chromosome number that is not a multiple of the haploid number. Most common class of aneuploidy being autosomal trisomy (60%) followed by monosomy X (20%). Trisomy 16 and trisomy 21 are overwhelmingly due to nondisjunction in meiosis I and have an exponential increase in incidence with increasing maternal age, particularly after age 35. In contrast, trisomy 18 is typically due to an error in meiosis II and shows a linear increase in incidence starting even before age 20. Environmental factors such as exposure to bisphenol A (BPA), an industrial chemical, can also increase the incidence of aneuploidy.

Polyploidy: The presence of a multiple of the haploid chromosome number other than two is the result of uniparental disomy (single chromosome or whole genome).

Parental chromosomal abnormalities: Translocations, inversions, and (rarely) ring chromosomes, are found in 3%–5% of couples with RPL compared with 0.2%–0.7% in the general population. Balanced translocations are the most common chromosomal abnormality contributing to RPL. Balanced translocations can be divided into reciprocal (60%) and Robertsonian (40%) translocations.

RCOG green top guideline 2023 states while quantitative fetal chromosomal abnormalities are the major cause of sporadic pregnancy loss, there is an inverse relationship with fetal aneuploidy and RPL presumably owing to the higher chance of a persistent maternal pathology rather than a sporadic aneuploidy. Equally, a finding of an aneuploid embryo has been found to confer an improved prognosis in the subsequent pregnancy.

Evidence gap: Polyploidy are lethal cytogenetic abnormalities which may be missed with array comparative genomic hybridization (aCGH) or traditional G-band karyotyping but can be detected with an SNP array, clinical application of which needs to be implored upon.

Q7. In what way can other causative genetic components be evaluated?

Draft recommendation: Few single-gene mutations causing pregnancy loss have been identified, and primarily associated with second-trimester losses. Identifying de novo mutations in the miscarried fetus or embryo often relies on technologies such as whole exome sequencing and whole genome sequencing.

Summary of evidence: A recessive but lethal syndrome would be unlikely to present as RPL because there would only be a 25% chance of the embryo inheriting both lethal copies of the gene and thus only a 1.6% chance of a homozygous lethal mutation being present in three consecutive pregnancies. An example of a recessive disorder responsible for fetal death at 14–20 weeks is lethal multiple pterygium syndrome, which presents with variable features such as hydrops and arthrogryposis.

However, lethal mutations may be more commonly found with X-linked conditions due to the single copy present in males and skewed X-inactivation. A number of X-linked male in utero lethal disorders have been identified, including Aicardi syndrome, chondrodysplasia punctata type 2, Goltz syndrome, incontinentia pigmenti, Rett syndrome, and oral-facial-digital syndrome type I.

ESHRE 2022 mentions next-generation sequencing (NGS) and whole exome sequencing (WES) as potential techniques for better detection of genetic components in RPL.

Evidence gap: Cost benefit analysis for implementation of whole exome sequencing (WES) to identify single gene disorders causing RPL needs to be carried out.

Q8. How may post-test genetic counseling be used to provide options for management for natural or assisted conception (IUI–IVF)?

Draft recommendation:

- Post-test genetic counseling is essential to inform couples of all of their reproductive and testing options and to educate them about the potential risks associated management options. If any of the parent is found to be a carrier of chromosomal translocation or a common dominant single gene variant or couple with carrier of identical variant or a female who is a carrier of X-linked disorder, prenatal diagnosis is offered to discuss the options of management.

- Options for couples with chromosomal rearrangements include attempting a further natural conception, preimplantation genetic testing (PGT), or gamete donation.
- Natural conception followed by prenatal genetic testing using amniocentesis, or chorionic villus sampling are options to detect the genetic abnormality in the offspring.
- Preimplantation genetic testing for structural rearrangements (PGT-SR) or preimplantation genetic testing for aneuploidy (PGT-A) can be carried out to select embryos not affected by parental chromosomal rearrangement or aneuploidy with transfer of unaffected embryos.

Summary of evidence:
ASRM 2012 suggests the above-mentioned treatment options.

RCOG green top guideline 2023 recommends there is insufficient data to support the routine use of PGT-A for couples with unexplained recurrent miscarriage. While the treatment may carry a significant cost, it may not improve the outcomes significantly.

Evidence gap: Observational studies have not demonstrated improved outcomes to date, both in terms of live birth rate and time to pregnancy interval with the routine use of PGT-A. RCTs are urgently required.

BIBLIOGRAPHY

1. Benson CB, Doubilet PM, Cooney MJ, et al. Early singleton pregnancy outcome: effects of maternal age and mode of conception. Radiology. 1997;203:399-403.
2. Deng TB, Liao XB, Zhu S. Recent advances in treatment of recurrent spontaneous abortion. Obstet Gynecol Surv. 2022;77:355-66.
3. Dimitriadis E, Menkhorst E, Saito S, et al. Recurrent pregnancy loss. Nat Rev Dis Prim. 2020;6:98.
4. ESHRE Recurrent Pregnancy Loss Guideline Development Group. Recurrent Pregnancy Loss: Guideline of European Society of Human Reproduction and Embryology. Strombeek-Bever: European Society of Human Reproduction and Embryology; 2022.
5. Gil-Villa AM, Cardona-Maya W, Agarwal A, et al. Assessment of sperm factors possibly involved in early recurrent pregnancy loss. Fertil Steril. 2010; 94(4):1465-72.
6. Hyde KJ, Schust DJ. Genetic considerations in recurrent pregnancy loss. Cold Spring Harb Perspect Med. 2015;5(3):a023119.
7. Li YH, Marren A. Recurrent pregnancy loss: a summary of international evidence-based guidelines and practice. Aust J Gen Pract. 2018;47:432-6.
8. Lilienthal D, Cahr M. Genetic counseling and assisted reproductive technologies. Cold Spring Harb Perspect Med. 2020;10(11):a036566.
9. Practice Committee of the American Society for Reproductive Medicine. Definitions of infertility and recurrent pregnancy loss: a committee opinion. Fertil Steril. 2013;99(1):63.

10. Practice Committee of the American Society for Reproductive Medicine. Evaluation and treatment of recurrent pregnancy loss: a committee opinion. Fertil Steril. 2012;98(5):1103-11.
11. Pylyp LY, Spynenko LO, Verhoglyad NV, et al. Chromosomal abnormalities in products of conception of first-trimester miscarriages detected by conventional cytogenetic analysis: a review of 1000 cases. J Assist Reprod Genet. 2018;35(2): 265-71.
12. Royal College of Obstetricians and Gynaecologists. Recurrent Miscarriage (Green-top Guideline No. 17). London: Royal College of Obstetricians and Gynaecologists; 2023.
13. Salat-Baroux J. Recurrent spontaneous abortions. Reprod Nutr Dev. 1988; 28(6B):1555-68.
14. Simpson JL, Mills JL, Holmes LB, et al. Low fetal loss rates after ultrasound-proved viability in early pregnancy. JAMA. 1987;256:2555-7.
15. Turesheva A, Aimagambetova G, Ukybassova T, et al. Recurrent pregnancy loss etiology, risk factors, diagnosis, and management. Fresh Look into a Full Box. J Clin Med. 2023;12:4074.

CHAPTER 11

Genetics and Hemoglobinopathies

Vandana Chaddha

Q1. What is the burden of *hemoglobinopathies* in Indian subcontinent? Should universal screening for hemoglobinopathy be performed in the Indian subcontinent? Why is it more clinically relevant to screen for β-thalassemia and β-thalassemia syndromes like sickle-cell anemia rather than α-thalassemia?

Draft recommendations:

- Keeping the burden of β-thalassemia universal screening for the same should be performed in the Indian subcontinent.
- Screening for α-thalassemia is not recommended.

Summary of evidence: The epidemiology of the hemoglobinopathies is a major factor informing decision-making regarding the screening approach. β-thalassemia is the most common single gene disorder in India. The carrier frequency of β-thalassemia in India ranges from 2 to 17% in different population with average frequency being 3%. Carriers can easily be diagnosed. Universal screening for the same should be performed in the Indian subcontinent.

β-thalassemia is an autosomal recessive disorder. Hence, if both the couple are carrier for it, then there is 25% risk of their child born with thalassemia major. The child becomes symptomatic with anemia after 4–6 months of life and remains transfusion dependent throughout life and needs iron chelation therapy. β-thalassemia in combination with sickle cell or HbE can produce the same clinical manifestation with lesser severity. To avoid having such an offspring or child, universal screening of prospective couple should be done. Moreover, Hb HPLC will also detect HbS and HbE along with carrier status of β-thalassemia, i.e., HbA2 simultaneously. No extra test needs to be done for the screening for other β-thalassemia syndromes. Whereas, β-thalassemia is manifested as anemia in infancy, α-thalassemia may present in intrauterine life as hydrops if all four α genes are absent and can be detected by USG.

Carrier frequencies in India:

- Prevalence of β-thalassemia carriers is 3–4%, Delhi: 5.5%; Mumbai: 2.7%; and Kolkata: 3.1%.

- Prevalence of α-thalassemia carriers: 13% (3–18%)
- Higher frequency in Sindhis, Punjabis, Gujaratis, Bengalis, Kolis, Mahars, Saraswats, Lohanas, and Gaurs
- HbS is more prevalent in the tribals of southern (Wynand district of Kerela), Central and Western states (Maharashtra, Gujarat, and Rajasthan) and reaching as high as 48% in some communities.
- HbE is more common in Northeastern states and has a carrier frequency of 50% in some areas.
- Lower HbD frequency in the eastern states of West Bengal is present in about 2% of people in Punjab.
- HbD seen in Punjab: 3–4%.
- *Summary of variants India:* HbD Punjab, HbD Iran, HbQ India, HbE, HbS, and HbC.

Global burden: Sickle-cell disease and thalassemia are among the most common genetic diseases worldwide. Globally, approximately 7% of pregnant individuals are heterozygous carriers of α- or β-thalassemia trait or hemoglobin (Hb) S, C, D Punjab, or E, and over 1% of couples are at risk of having an affected child.

- *Carrier frequency for hemoglobinopathies:* 1–20%
- Every year 300,000–400,000 babies are born with β-thalassemia major.
- Mediterranean basin, Middle East, parts of Africa, Indian subcontinent, and Southeast Asia have higher prevalence.

Unlike β-thalassemia, α-thalassemia produces intrauterine disease and will be detected on USG, so β-thalassemia will be the more clinically relevant condition to screen.

Research gap: The incidence varies by different areas in the country and may be underreported in resource-limited communities where diagnostic testing is not routinely available. Population migration and interethnic marriages are on the rise in India and may present challenging new combinations of thalassemia syndromes in couples.

Q2. Which are the major *asymptomatic* carriers, compound heterozygotes, homozygous states of β-globin gene and α-globin gene found in India? What are the combinations of hemoglobin variants in carrier parents which will not require prenatal testing?

Draft recommendations: Major *asymptomatic* carriers, compound heterozygotes, homozygous states of β-globin gene and α-globin gene found in India are:

1	Carrier-β-thalassemia trait
2	Carrier-HbS trait
3	Carrier-HbE trait
4	Carrier-HbD trait
5	Carrier-δ-β-thalassemia trait
6	Carrier-Hb Lepore
7	Carrier-HPFH trait
8	Compound Heterozygote for HbD and HbE
9	Compound heterozygote for HbS and HbE (βS/βE)
10	Compound heterozygote for HbS and HPFH (βS/HPFH)
11	Compound heterozygote βT/HbD—common referral from North India
12	Homozygous HbD (βD/βD)
13	Homozygous HbE (βE/βE) common referral from Northeast

Q3. Which are the major *symptomatic* homozygous/compound heterozygous states of β-globin gene found in India? What are the combinations of hemoglobin variants in carrier parents which will definitely require prenatal testing?

Draft recommendations: Major *symptomatic* homozygous/compound heterozygous states of β-globin gene found in India are:

1	βT/βT (includes β0/β0, β0/β+ and β+/β+ genotypes)—PND offered
2	βT/βE (HbE)—PND offered
3	βT/sickle-severe—PND offered
4	βE/βE (HbE)—PND offered
5	Sickle trait/sickle trait—PND offered
6	βT/HbLepore—PND offered
7	βT/δβ—PND offered
8	βT/HPFH—PND offered

βT—indicating a β-thalassemia mutant allele
Beta0 variants: Abolish β-globin production
Beta+ variants: These can produce some β-globin but far less than the normal amount
Source: (ACOG 2022) (National health mission guidelines, 2016)

Research gap: More data needed for genotype phenotype correlation of various thalassemia syndromes to distinguish between thalassemia major and intermedia to give informed choices to couple considering prenatal diagnosis and termination of pregnancy. The severity of sickle-cell disease in India is reported to be less and the etiology needs further research.

Q4. Should complete blood count (CBC) be performed as an adjunct to high-performance liquid chromatography (HPLC) for thalassemia carrier screening? What are the classical blood indices in parents with carrier status of β-thalassemia? What is a silent carrier and what would be the test of choice for detection of the same?

Draft recommendations and evidence:

All pregnant patients should have a *complete blood count (CBC)—including MCV and/or MCH should be performed along with Hb HPLC.*

- Easy to perform
- Readily available in countries with limited resources
- Provides baseline hemoglobin/hematocrit.
- Can detect iron-deficiency anemia which is more prevalent in India.

Beta-thalassemia trait will have MCV < 80 femtoliters (fL), MCH < 27 picogram (pg) and HbA2 > 3.5%.

Maternal hemoglobin analysis that can be performed by protein chemistry methods include:

- Capillary electrophoresis
- Isoelectric focusing
- Hemoglobin electrophoresis
- *High-performance liquid chromatography (HPLC)*

These "first-line" hematological and protein chemistry tests (HPLC) will detect most common hemoglobinopathies.

Silent carrier: Atypical β-thalassemia trait cases the percentage of HbA2 and HbF are not elevated, so these carriers will be missed on HPLC testing and are called silent carrier. Iron deficiency, particularly when severe (estimated at ferritin level less than 15 ng/mL), should be corrected and retesting to be done. If timely correction is not possible, DNA-based testing can be performed since results are independent of iron status.

The European Network for Rare and Congenital Anemias (ENERCA) recommends that carrier detection should be mandatory with current hematological and protein chemistry tests. However, DNA analysis should be applied in complex cases or when results to these initial tests are unclear.

B-globin gene sequencing would be the test of choice for detection of silent carriers.

Research gap: Acceptability of universal screening and its effectiveness including cost-effective analysis is not studied in India.

Q5. When is DNA-based testing typically performed? What is NGS-based testing?

Draft recommendations:

DNA-based confirmatory tests are typically performed when:

- First-line screening test results are abnormal *or* ambiguous (e.g., microcytosis with normal iron study)

- The patient has normal first-line screening test results but epidemiologic or familial risk suggest β-thalassemia carrier status (e.g., previous history of thalassemia major child requiring repeated blood transfusion)
- The pregnancy is at an advanced gestational age where definitive diagnosis needs to be achieved rapidly for pregnancy management.
- Knowledge of the exact variant(s) can assist in predicting the clinical phenotype and discussing it with the prospect parent(s).
- Previous history of nonimmune hydrops fetalis without any other cause

Various DNA-based tests available are:

- *ARMS-PCR:* It looks into specific mutation that is prevalent in the ethnic group. After the easy availability of β-globin gene sequencing, this is rarely used.
- *Beta-globin gene sequencing:* It looks into mutation present in β-globin gene and the most reliable method.
- *Next generation sequencing (NGS):* In addition to the mutation in β-globin gene, it also looks into any clinically relevant mutation in other genes including α-globin gene.

Summary of evidence:

New screening approaches: Next generation sequencing (NGS) methodology is a promising investigational approach for universal screening because of high sensitivity for carrier detection and ability to detect new variants).

In a Chinese population that was not ethnically diverse, a large-scale premarital carrier screening program for α-and β-thalassemia reported a higher thalassemia carrier rate using NGS screening compared with the traditional approach (i.e., RBC indices combined with hemoglobin electrophoresis and subsequent genotyping of screen positives by gap-PCR and reverse dot blot hybridization or sequencing; 49.5 vs. 22%). Another study of the traditional prepregnancy approach among 944 couples in China reported that it had lower sensitivity and a higher missed diagnosis ratio (61 and 39%, respectively) for α-thalassemia variants compared with NGS combined with gap-PCR aimed to detect deletions known to be responsible for 80% of the molecular causes of α-thalassemia.

Research gap: The benefit of NGS over the conventional DNA analysis and its utility in Indian population is yet to be studied.

Q6. What is the most essential prerequisite for prenatal diagnosis of thalassemia?

Draft recommendations and evidence: (ACOG, 2022), (National health mission guidelines, 2016]

- Identify pregnant individuals at risk of having a fetus with hemoglobinopathy.
- Parental mutations should be done before hand.

- Counseling regarding the risks, limitations, and benefits of testing
- Informed decision on whether to proceed with fetal genetic testing and should understand how the results of genetic testing will impact their reproductive choices.
- Consider ethical considerations and the cultural and social background of the individual and their family in the Pretest counseling. Identify Rh negative mothers for anti-D prophylaxis.
- Informed written consents as per the local laws. CVS is ideal for molecular diagnosis.
- Mutation analysis should be done only once.
- Emphasize that autosomal recessive conditions have a 25% recurrence risk in each pregnancy and prenatal testing needs to be done in each pregnancy.

Q7. What is the invasive procedure of choice for prenatal diagnosis of thalassemia?

Draft recommendations:

- *Chorionic villus sampling:* When gestational age is 11–14 weeks
- *Amniocentesis:* At gestational age after 16 weeks
- *Cordocentesis:* At late gestation

Summary of evidence: DNA-based testing for thalassemia can be performed during the first trimester of pregnancy on villi obtained by chorionic villus sampling (CVS, which is typically done at 11–14 weeks of gestation) or on cells in amniotic fluid obtained by amniocentesis (typically performed at ≥15 weeks of gestation).

If patients present at late gestation and mutation analysis has not been done, FBS is a better option as HPLC can be done on the cord blood and one gets more time to identify mutation.

Research gap: Ultrasound-guided aspiration of celomic fluid is an investigational technique for very early prenatal diagnosis of hemoglobinopathy when in utero intervention is being considered.

Q8. Is NIPT commercially available for prenatal diagnosis of thalassemia syndromes?

Draft recommendations: NIPT is not commercially offered for thalassemia testing.

Summary of evidence: Noninvasive screening is an alternative to an invasive procedure for diagnostic testing, but the sensitivity and specificity for hemoglobinopathies have not been established. It is considered investigational because the methodology has more challenges than aneuploidy screening for the common trisomies and sex chromosome aneuploidies.

Research gap: Lack of adequate validation studies.

Q9. Is preimplantation genetic mutation testing a viable option to prevent thalassemia major?

Draft recommendations: Preimplantation genetic testing for monogenic disorders (PGT-M) to identify affected and unaffected embryos in vitro can be performed successfully in couples who are thalassemia heterozygotes or sickle cell heterozygotes or homozygotes and willing to undergo IVF with preimplantation genetic diagnosis. It needs to be emphasized that a confirmatory prenatal diagnosis testing is recommended even after that.

Summary of evidence: Diagnostic accuracy is >99%. This procedure can only be performed in conjunction with in vitro fertilization (IVF). Couples may choose to undergo IVF with PGT and transfer of embryos unlikely to be affected by hemoglobinopathy, thereby avoiding the need to consider termination or potentially morbid in-utero and postnatal therapy of an affected pregnancy. Confirmatory prenatal diagnostic testing is recommended.

Research gap: Inadvertent amplification of contaminating extraneous DNA can lead to false-negative results and transfer of abnormal embryos thought to be normal. Errors in PGT-M can also result when one allele for the gene of interest fails to amplify ("allele drop-out") or amplifies poorly ("partial amplification"). Both types of technical failure have been described and have resulted in misdiagnoses leading to the transfer of an affected embryo believed to be normal or the discarding of a normal embryo thought to be affected.

Summary

- Prevention is the key to the management of hemoglobinopathies.
- Screen every couple/woman who presents in the preconception or prenatal settings.
- Family history is important for cascade screening.
- *CBC with peripheral smear:* MCV < 75 and MCH < 25.
- Hb electrophoresis/HPLC/Sickling tests if HbS/D
- *HPLC-A2 > 3.5%:* Screen partner
- Prenatal diagnosis should be offered if both partners are carriers.
- *Mutation study:* Sequencing/NGS promising new technique
- Mutation identification of the couple should be in place before invasive testing is done.
- Population-based NGS screening for hemoglobinopathies may be more advantageous specially in Far eastern countries with higher load of α-thalassemia.

BIBLIOGRAPHY

1. Achour A, Koopmann TT, Baas F, et al. The evolving role of next-generation sequencing in screening and diagnosis of hemoglobinopathies. Front Physiol. 2021;12:686689.

2. Adamski C, Terhaar C, DaRe J, et al. Hemoglobinopathy evaluation in routine carrier testing: results to inform guidelines and protocols. Obstet Gynecol. 2019;133:163.
3. American College of Obstetricians and Gynecologists Practice Advisory. (2022). Hemoglobinopathies in Pregnancy. [online] Available from https://www.acog.org/clinical/clinical-guidance/practice-advisory/articles/2022/08/hemoglobinopathies-in-pregnancy. [Last accessed November, 2024].
4. Erlich HA, López-Peña C, Carlberg KT, et al. Noninvasive Prenatal Test for β-Thalassemia and Sickle Cell Disease Using Probe Capture Enrichment and Next-Generation Sequencing of DNA in Maternal Plasma. J Appl Lab Med. 2022;7:515.
5. He J, Song W, Yang J, et al. Next-generation sequencing improves thalassemia carrier screening among premarital adults in a high prevalence population: the Dai nationality, China. Genet Med. 2017;19:1022
6. Kuliev A, Rechitsky S, Verlinsky O, et al. Preimplantation diagnosis and HLA typing for haemoglobin disorders. Reprod Biomed Online. 2005;11:362.
7. Ministry of Health and Family Welfare Government of India. National Health Mission Guidelines on Hemoglobinopathies in India. New Delhi: Ministry of Health and Family Welfare; 2016.
8. Mohanty D, Colah RB, Gorakshakar AC, et al. Prevalence of β-thalassemia and other haemoglobinopathies in six cities in India: a multicentre study. 2013;4(1):33-42.
9. Piel FB. The present and future global burden of the inherited disorders of hemoglobin. Hematol Oncol Clin North Am. 2016;30:327.
10. Thammavong K, Luewan S, Wanapirak C, et al. Ultrasound features of fetal anemia lessons from hemoglobin bart disease. J Ultrasound Med. 2021; 40:659.
11. Traeger-Synodinos J, Harteveld CL, Old JM, et al. EMQN Best Practice Guidelines for molecular and haematology methods for carrier identification and prenatal diagnosis of the haemoglobinopathies. Eur J Hum Genet. 2015;23:426.
12. Zhao J, Li J, Lai Q, et al. Combined use of gap-PCR and next-generation sequencing improves thalassaemia carrier screening among premarital adults in China. J Clin Pathol. 2020;73:488.

CHAPTER 12

Applications of Molecular Genetic Technologies to Prenatal Diagnosis

Parag M Tamhankar, Vasundhara P Tamhankar, Shalin S Vaniawala

Q1. What is chromosomal microarray?

Draft recommendations: Chromosomal microarray is a chip-based method to determine chromosomal aneuploidies, polyploidies, microdeletions (submicroscopic losses of chromosomal material), and microduplications (submicroscopic gains of chromosomal material). Thus, this is a technology that identifies copy number variants of chromosomal material or genes. It can detect monosomy, trisomy, triploidy, common and rare microdeletion, and duplication syndromes.

Types of microarray include:

- Bacterial artificial chromosome clone (BAC) arrays and
- Single nucleotide polymorphism probe (SNP) arrays. SNP arrays can additionally detect regions of loss of heterozygosity (homozygous regions of chromosome that share the same SNPs over a long stretch) which help detect imprinting disorders due to uniparental disomy (both chromosomes from single parent) and mapping of autosomal recessive disorders in consanguineous families.
    - The resolution of microarray depends on the probe density. For example, an Affymetrix 315K chipset has a resolution of 1 megabase (1,000 kilobase) for deletions and 2 megabase (2,000 kilobase) for duplications.
    - The size of the copy number variant does not determine its pathogenicity. It is determined by the content of genes in the region of interest. The genes known to be sensitive to haploinsufficiency (deletion of one copy) should be included in pathogenic microdeletion syndromes and genes known to be sensitive for triploinsufficiency (presence of three copies of gene) should be included in pathogenic microduplication syndromes.

Q2. What are the indications and limitations of chromosomal microarray?

Draft recommendations:

- The primary indication of microarray in prenatal diagnosis is structural anomalies in the fetus such as congenital heart defect, bilateral club foot, arthrogryposis, diaphragmatic hernia, cerebral ventriculomegaly or hydrocephalus, omphalocele, cleft lip and palate, micrognathia, neural tube defect, microcephaly or brain malformations such as pachygyria, Dandy Walker malformation, agenesis/hypoplasia of corpus callosum, Arnold Chiari malformation, short limbs, cystic kidneys, cystic hygroma, fetal hydrops, unexplained still birth or intrauterine fetal death, etc.

- *Previous child with autism or intellectual disability:* Diagnosis in index child and segregation analysis of the variant in parents is essential to provide definitive prenatal diagnosis. The chance on microarray abnormality in autism spectrum disorder with or without intellectual abnormality is reported to be 10–20%.
- Microarray can be an alternative to fetal karyotype in case of invasive testing being performed for single gene disorder in a structurally normal fetus; for example, using microarray concurrent to the prenatal diagnosis of beta thalassemia by HBB gene sequencing. If the fetus is found to be unaffected, then microarray may be done to rule out common aneuploidy like trisomy 21.

Limitations: The limitations of microarray are as follows.

- Mosaicism <20% cannot be detected in microarray.
- Also, structural chromosome changes such as balanced translocation or inversion or ring chromosomes cannot be detected on microarray. These can only be detected on karyotyping.
- The type of trisomy whether it is nondisjunction/translocation type cannot be determined.
- Triploidy may not be picked up on certain types of microarray.
- Uniparental disomy can also be detected on microarray, however, parent of origin of the chromosome cannot be determined. For example, uniparental disomy of chromosome 11 can lead to either Beckwith Wiedemann syndrome or Russell Silver syndrome. However, identifying the correct diagnosis will require methylation sensitive multiplex ligation dependent probe amplification (MS-MLPA) method **(Fig 1)**.

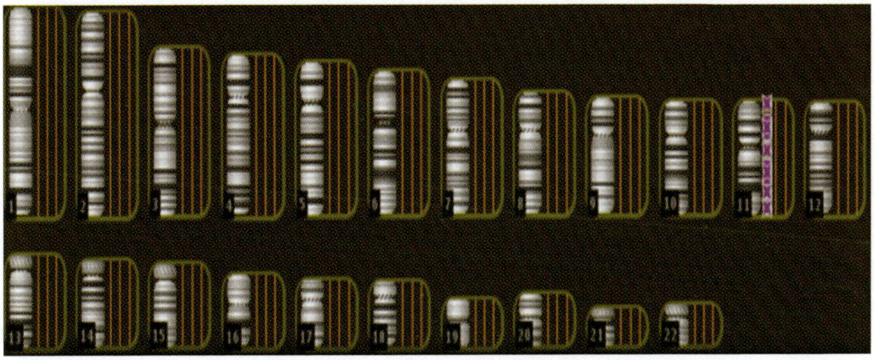

Fig. 1: Uniparental disomy of chromosome 11.

Summary of evidence: The ACOG Committee opinion (2016) gives the guidelines on use of microarray and NGS in prenatal practice. It quotes the study by Wapner et al. 2012, which showed that microarray identified all the aneuploidies and unbalanced translocations diagnosed by a karyotype and gave an additional yield of clinically significant abnormalities in 6% cases with abnormal USG and normal karyotype. Microarrays could detect an abnormality in 1.7% cases with normal USG and normal karyotype. Wapner et al. 2012, also showed that for fetuses with structural abnormalities, the diagnostic yield is approximately 49% in first trimester and 17% in second trimester. In the study by Xia et al. 2020, microarrays could detect abnormalities in 3.8% more cases than karyotype analysis. The organ systems associated with abnormal microarray results are cardiac, urogenital, central nervous system, and skeletal. Isolated cardiac and renal malformations show an incremental yield of 15% and 10.6% over karyotype, respectively. Isolated cardiac outflow tract anomalies have an incremental yield of 30% (Donnelly et al. 2014). In postnatal cases, microarray has an additional diagnostic yield over karyotype of 12–15% in cases of congenital malformations, developmental delay, or intellectual disability. Shaffer et al. (2001), Eggerman et al. (2016), and Wang et al. (2019) note that most cases of uniparental disomy do not give any phenotypic abnormalities. However, maternal UPD of 2, 7, 11, 14, and 15 and paternal UPD of 6, 11, 15, and 20 could lead to imprinting disorders leading to abnormalities in growth and development of the child.

Research gap/limitation: There is not a uniform classification for several microdeletion/duplication syndromes. For example, the 15q11.2 BP1-BP2 microdeletion syndrome (Burnside Butler syndrome) which includes genes *NIPA1, NIPA2, CYFIP1,* and *TUBGCP5* has been denoted as pathogenic for developmental delay/autism by some studies whereas other studies denote the deletion as likely benign. There is no general consensus on reporting such variants.

In certain cases, the penetrance can be variable. For example, the proximal 16p11.2 deletion syndrome which includes *PRRT2* gene can be extremely variable, ranging from autism, intellectual disability, epilepsy to normal phenotype.

Q3. How do we interpret or read the chromosomal microarray report?

The standard format of results obtained on chromosomal microarray is given as follows:

Example 1: Report: arr(GRCh37)(1-22)x2,(XY or XX)x1. This can be decoded as follows:

i. arr denotes microarray
ii. GRCh37 denotes GRCh37 Genome Reference Consortium Human Build 37 (GRCh37).

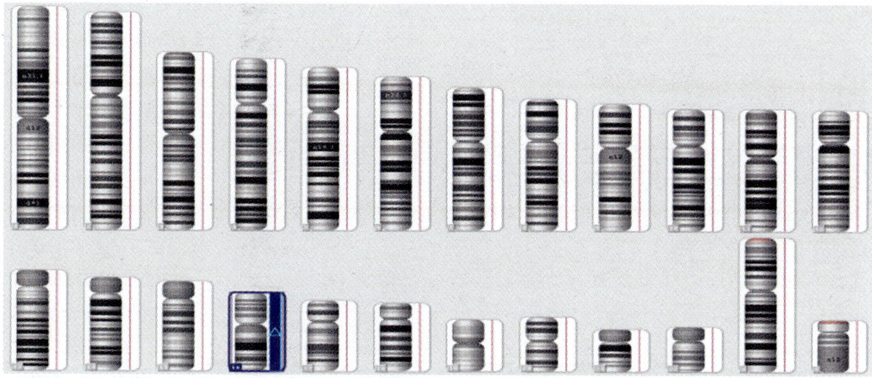

Fig. 2: Karyoview showing Trisomy 16.

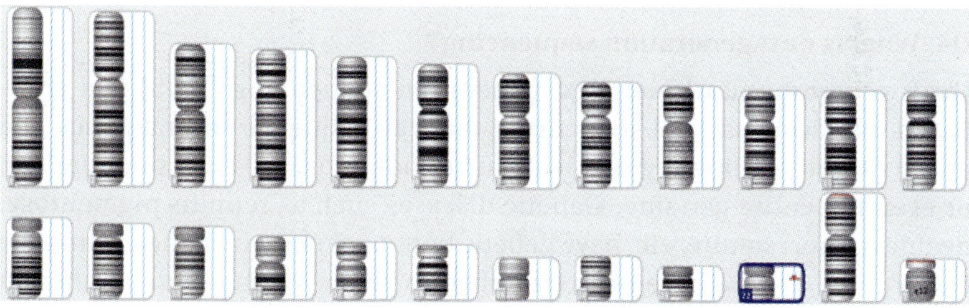

Fig. 3: Karyoview showing 22q11.2 deletion syndrome and detailed chromosomal view of chromosome 22 showing the deletion.

iii. (1-22)x2 denotes normal two copies of each autosome, and
iv. XY denotes normal male chromosomes with normal one copy each of X and Y chromosome.

Example 2: Trisomy 16 can be mentioned as arr(GRCh37)16p13.3q24.3 (85,881_90,155,062) x 3 which shows that there are a 90,069 kilobases from cytoband 16p13.3 to 16q24.3 (tip of p arm to tip of q arm of chromosome 16) extra **(Fig. 2)**.

Example 3: DiGeorge syndrome or 22q11.2 deletion syndrome, a common syndromic cause for congenital heart disease is written as arr(GRCh37) 22q11.21(18,917,031_21,465,662) x 1. This indicates deletion of 2,549 kilobases of chromosomal material on chromosome 22 on cytoband q11.21 which includes 75 genes **(Fig. 3)**.

Example 4: Triploidy can be detected by noting the allele difference segment which shows four lines instead of the normal three (ACOG, 2016) **(Fig. 4)**.

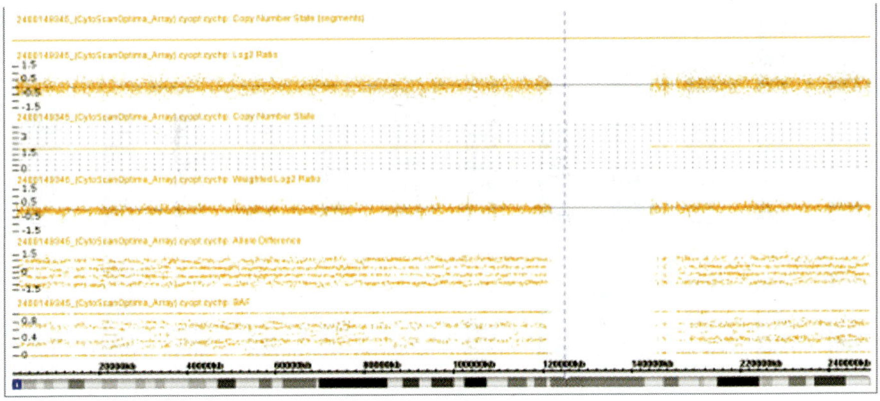

Fig. 4: Chromosome detail view with Allele difference segment showing four lines denoting triploidy. Maternal cell contamination will also show similar pattern.

Q4. What is next generation sequencing?

Draft recommendations: Next-generation sequencing (NGS) is a chip-based massively parallel sequencing that can sequence several genes, the entire exome (coding regions with surrounding intron–exon boundaries), or even the entire genome. Genetic diseases such as retinitis pigmentosa, deafness, short stature, etc. have genetic heterogeneity which means that the cause of the disease have been identified to be due to mutation in different genes. It is cumbersome to sequence several genes one by one. NGS is used to identify the variants in such cases. This technology has revolutionized modern medicine and has made molecular diagnosis of genetic syndromes possible and affordable to the masses.

Q5. What are the indications and limitations of next generation sequencing?

Draft recommendations: The *prenatal indications* of exome sequencing or NGS sequencing are fetal anomalies such as polycystic kidney disease, cystic hygroma, hydrops fetalis, fetal skeletal dysplasias, fetal neural tube defects, polyhydramnios, cerebral ventriculomegaly, agenesis/hypoplasia of corpus callosum, hydrocephalus, fetal brain malformations, Binder facies, limb anomalies, spine anomalies, cleft lip/palate, bilateral talipes equinovarus, arthrogryposis multiplex, diaphragmatic hernia, congenital heart defect, intrauterine growth retardation, etc.

The *postnatal indications* of exome sequencing is diagnosis of idiopathic mental retardation, autism, other neurodevelopmental syndromes such as primary microcephaly, pachygyria-lissencephaly and other brain malformation syndromes, genodermatoses such as ichthyosis, epidermolysis bullosa, photosensitive dermatoses, xeroderma pigmentosum, dyskeratosis congenita, liver diseases such as cholestatic syndromes, cirrhosis, neurodegenerative conditions such as Rett syndrome, leukodystrophies, dystonia, dementia, ataxia, Parkinsonism, kidney diseases such as cystic kidney disease, glomerular diseases, nephrotic syndromes, tubulointerstitial diseases, skeletal dysplasias such as rhizomelic dysplasia, mesomelic dysplasia, acromelic dysplasias, lethal skeletal dysplasias, short rib syndromes, platyspondylic syndromes, spondyloepi-metaphyseal dysplasias, achondrogenesis, osteogenesis imperfecta, craniosynostosis syndromes, osteopetrosis and other increased bone density syndromes, ocular diseases such as retinitis pigmentosa, Lebers congenital amaurosis, congenital cataract, anterior segment dysgenesis, corneal dystrophies, optic neuropathy, oculocutaneous albinism, cardiac conditions such as cardiomyopathies, cardiac arrhythmias, Brugada syndrome, long QT syndrome, congenital heart defects, hematological conditions such as hemoglobinopathies, aplastic anemia, bone marrow diseases, immunological conditions such as primary immunodeficiency, hypogammaglobulinemia, combined immunodeficiency syndromes, hemophagocytic syndromes, lymphoproliferative syndromes, inborn errors of metabolism such as amino acidopathies, organic acidemia, urea cycle disorders, peroxisomal disorders, lysosomal storage disorders, glycogen storage disorders, mitochondrial disorders, deafness, hereditary cancer syndromes, etc.

Diagnosis in index case and parental analysis is essential for a definitive diagnosis, recurrence risk assessment, and definitive prenatal diagnosis. The diagnostic yield of solo exome sequencing in case of fetal anomalies is around 30% whereas exome trio (fetus plus parents) has a yield of around 35%. Exome sequencing can also provide copy number variants such as microdeletions and microduplications using bioinformatic tools. Hence, this technology is proven to complement high resolution microarray/MLPA in diagnosis of copy number variants.

Prenatal diagnosis can be provided for childhood onset cancers such as retinoblastoma and can be avoided for adult-onset cancer susceptibility conditions with incomplete penetrance such as colon cancer, breast cancer, and ovarian cancer. Unwarranted medical termination of pregnancy for treatable adult-onset cancer susceptibility with incomplete penetrance can thus be avoided. Preimplantation genetic diagnosis for such conditions will be a more ethical way.

Summary of evidence: Mellis et al. (2022) conducted a review of 72 reports from 66 studies representing 4,350 fetuses to determine the yield of exome in cases of fetal structural anomalies wherein microarray and karyotype was normal. The pooled incremental yield of exome sequencing was 31%. In case where Mendelian etiology was suspected on USG/clinical history, the yield of exome sequencing was higher (42% in Mendelian etiology selected cases over 15% in unselected cases). The pooled incremental diagnostic yield of exome sequencing over microarray was 53% in skeletal cases, 37% in neuromuscular cases/fetal akinesia, 29% in multisystem cases, 22% in hydrops/edema, 17% in central nervous system anomalies, 11% in cardiac anomalies, 9% in craniofacial anomalies, 4% in fetal growth restriction, and 2% in isolated increase in nuchal translucency. Prenatal exome sequencing showed an additional yield of 31% wherein microarray and karyotype were normal.

The limitation of NGS is as follows:

- It cannot diagnose chromosomal rearrangements such as translocations, inversions, ring chromosome, etc.
- It cannot be used to diagnose tritetra or penta nucleotide repeat expansion disorders such as fragile X, spinocerebellar ataxia, Friedreich ataxia, *DMPK* gene-related myotonic dystrophy, Huntington disease, etc.
- NGS cannot reliably diagnose disorders that are related to genes that have a related pseudogene. For example, *CYP21A2* gene-related congenital adrenal hyperplasia, *SMN1* gene related spinal muscular atrophy, *GBA* gene-related Gaucher disease. Deletion–duplication analysis such as MLPA (multiplex probe dependent probe amplification) and Sanger sequencing or PCR-based amplification of whole/partial gene followed by NGS is used for analysis of these genes.
- Also, the variants obtained in NGS should be confirmed by Sanger sequencing to rule out false positive variants in NGS. False positive variants may arise in nucleotide repeat regions, homopolymer stretches, AT or GC-rich regions, regions complex to sequence, or genes with pseudogenes.
- Heterozygous copy number variants involving single exons have a lower diagnostic yield by NGS than the *MLPA/QFPCR* for the same gene.

Research gap: The utility of NGS in indications such as identifying soft markers in pregnancy, maternal serum screening showing a risk for aneuploidy, and noninvasive prenatal screening showing a high risk for aneuploidy or microdeletion/duplication is not proven.

Reproductive decisions such as medical termination of pregnancy based on variants of uncertain significance are not recommended.

Similarly, prenatal diagnosis cannot be provided for complex disorders or in disorders due to genetic predisposition rather than causation such as type I or type II diabetes, *SPINK1* gene related recurrent pancreatitis, *ABCA7* gene related Alzheimer disease, *UGT1A1* gene related Gilbert syndrome, factor V Leiden heterozygosity for thrombophilia, *APOE* gene related hyperlipidemia, *MTHFR* gene c.677C>T polymorphism, *HLA-B27* associated ankylosing spondylitis, etc. Prenatal diagnosis for class II to class

IV variants of G6PD deficiency can be avoided since these do not cause chronic hemolytic anemia but confer risk of acute hemolysis on exposure to certain drugs or toxins which can be minimized by lifelong avoidance of these agents.

Prenatal diagnosis for late nontreatable, disabling adult-onset conditions such as Huntington disease, myotonic dystrophy, spinocerebellar ataxia, early onset Alzheimer disease (*PSEN1, PSEN2,* and *APP* genes), familial Parkinson disease, etc. can be possible in case parents wish to exercise their reproductive choice of discontinuation of pregnancy in case of an affected fetus. However, in case, parents are planning to continue the pregnancy even if the fetus is affected, the genetic diagnosis of the unborn child is suggested to be deferred respecting the fetus/individual autonomy. (Hercher et al., 2016). Similarly, there has been a debate over prenatal diagnosis of conditions such as nonsyndromic genetic deafness. The most common being *GJB2* gene related sensorineural deafness which can be treated successfully by cochlear transplant. Evidence from studies suggests that termination of pregnancy of an affected fetus with deafness or embryonic selection by PGD can be allowed if parents choose to do so.

Q6. How are genetic variants classified?

Draft recommendations: Genetic variants are to be classified into five categories: benign, likely benign, pathogenic, likely pathogenic, and variants of uncertain significance.

1 and 2. Benign and likely benign variants account for the normal phenotypic variation in the population. They are also called polymorphisms.

3. Pathogenic variants are well-established and accepted causative variants of a disease.
4. Likely pathogenic variants are novel variants with a high possibility of disease causation.
5. Variants of uncertain significance are variants with insufficient evidence of either disease causation or their benign nature. They could be reclassified into either benign or pathogenic in the future as more evidence is available.

Evidence: American College of Medical Genetics classifies genetic variants into five categories: Benign, likely benign, pathogenic, likely pathogenic, and variants of uncertain significance.

The criteria used to classify these variants include:

1. Nature of the variant, for example, variants such as nonsense variants, initiation codon variant, consensus splice site variant are very strong evidence of pathogenicity of a variant in a gene where loss of function is a known mechanism of disease,

2. Frequency of the variant in public genomic databases such as gnomAD, EXAC, etc.
3. *Evidence in published literature:* Same variant as a previously established pathogenic variant or benign variant; well established in-vitro or in-vivo functional studies demonstrate pathogenicity or benign nature, well established case-control studies or cohort studies demonstrating the variant effect.
4. Segregation pattern in affected and unaffected individuals in the family of the index case.
5. Multiple lines of computational evidence (insilico analysis) show pathogenic effect or benign nature.
6. Patients phenotype is highly specific for a genetic disease related to the gene described, for example, novel *RPE65* gene variant in retinitis pigmentosa.
7. Inheritance pattern of the variant observed in the family is known/not known to be associated with the disease concerned, for example, if a novel variant in *CDKL5* gene in a patient with Rett syndrome is present in an asymptomatic parent, then this shows evidence that the variant is likely benign since penetrance of *CDKL5* gene variants for Rett syndrome is known to be complete.

Research gap/limitation: Clinvar database is a representative database of ACMG classification of genomic variants https://www.ncbi.nlm.nih.gov/clinvar/. However, many variants have conflicting interpretations of pathogenicity. Also, classification of certain variants can change over time. Each laboratory must maintain its database regarding the internal frequency of rare variants, and the occurrence of the same variant in cases with similar presentation/disease, and make an effort to publish these variants and their presentations. It is also possible that variants may be reclassified depending on the segregation pattern of variants in the family members and the latest research publications about the variant. There is lack of coordinated effort among laboratories to maintain these databases owing to privacy/copyright and other concerns.

Q7. What are incidental findings in exome sequencing?

Draft recommendations: Incidental findings are variants in genes related to diseases/conditions that do not fit the primary indication/symptoms for which the exome sequencing was ordered.

We recommend reporting variants in genes related to medically treatable/actionable fetal/childhood or adult conditions as incidental findings, after obtaining patient consent in pretest counseling.

Evidence: In the paper by Miller et al., 2023, the ACMG recommends few medically actionable conditions/diseases can be added to the report after proper counseling with the patient and discussion with the referring clinician.

In addition to these genes, we also recommend reporting variants in the 409 genes included in the BabyDetect screening program especially while reporting exomes in neonates/infants/children after discussing with the family and referring clinician. (*Reference:* https://babydetect.com/en/pannel-v1-english/).

Some of the conditions are adult onset and a positive NGS report can initiate surveillance for these tumors/cancers/conditions. Lifestyle modifications can be suggested. Patients with long QT syndrome can be provided a list of drugs to avoid, and can be prescribed β-blockers to avoid arrhythmias.

However, there is a debate over the issue of incidental findings while reporting in prenatal settings. The ACMG and Canadian College of Medical Geneticists recommend that only pathogenic/likely pathogenic variants for fetal/ childhood onset can be considered whereas adult-onset conditions should not be reported. Whereas a Joint Position Statement from the International Society for Prenatal Diagnosis (ISPD), the Society for Maternal Fetal Medicine (SMFM), and the Perinatal Quality Foundation (PQF) addresses incidental findings in the context of prenatal genetic screening, recognizes that some laboratories may choose to report pathogenic and likely pathogenic variants in genes that lead to childhood- and adult-onset conditions, and suggest this topic should be covered during genetic counseling.

Research gap/limitations: There are no studies on the impact of incidental findings, in prenatal settings, on the affected families in the Indian context.

Q8. What is Sanger sequencing?

Draft recommendations: Sanger sequencing, also known as chain termination method of sequencing or di-deoxy sequencing, has been the mainstay of conventional part-by-part or exon-by-exon sequencing of the gene since its discovery in the 1970s. It can be used to sequence around 1,000 basepairs of nucleotides at a time of a targeted region of the gene. Since, the advent of NGS sequencing, genetic testing of large genes has shifted to NGS from Sanger sequencing since it is quicker and cost effective. However, Sanger sequencing is important for several indications.

Q9. What are the indications and limitations of Sanger sequencing?

Draft recommendations: The applications for sanger sequencing include the following.

- Sequencing of *HBB* gene in β-thalassemia, sickle-cell disease, and related hemoglobinopathies, targeted sequencing for common mutations such as *p.G380R* mutation in *FGFR3* gene in achondroplasia, *p.G608G* mutation in *LMNA* gene in Hutchinson Gilford progeria.

- Confirmation of sequence variant obtained in *NGS*. This validates the variant obtained in the index patient and can also be used for segregation pattern analysis in the family and affected and unaffected relatives.
- Genes that have a pseudogene can be amplified by long-range PCR and thereby subjected to Sanger sequencing. Examples include *SMN1* gene sequencing for spinal muscular atrophy, *ABCD1* gene sequencing for adrenoleukodystrophy, *CYP21A2* gene sequencing for 21 hydroxylase gene-related congenital adrenal hyperplasia, *GBA* gene sequencing for Gaucher disease.
- Prenatal diagnosis for familial mutation by Sanger sequencing, the known familial variant can be detected in fetal DNA by Sanger sequencing.

Evidence: In their papers on prenatal diagnosis by Lord et al. (2019), Fu et al. (2022), and Wang et al. (2024) all phenotypically relevant variants detected on exome sequencing were validated by Sanger sequencing. Sabath et al. (2017) reviewed all the diagnostic methods of diagnosis of β-thalassemia and noted that Sanger sequencing of *HBB* gene was one of the best methods of detecting point variants in *HBB* gene. However, it needed to be complimented by *MLPA* to detect deletions for a comprehensive coverage of all variants. They note that next generation sequencing-based methods have the capability to detect both point variants and deletions.

Limitations: The limitations of Sanger sequencing are as follows:

- *Allele dropout phenomenon:* The PCR may preferentially amplify only one allele thereby missing the variant on the other allele. This can be minimized by using two different sets of primers for PCR.
- Variants positive on NGS but negative on Sanger sequencing may mean false positive variant in NGS, low-grade mosaicism (variants present in <20% cells), or allele dropout phenomenon. Low-grade mosaicism can be diagnosed by increasing the depth of the sequencing panel.

Q10. What is a polymerase chain reaction?

Draft recommendations: Polymerase chain reaction (PCR) is a nucleic acid amplification technique used to identify a part of a gene of interest. It is a first step toward sequencing the nucleotide code of a gene.

Q11. What are the applications and limitations of polymerase chain reaction?

Draft recommendations: It can be used in the following instances in prenatal diagnosis.

ARMS PCR: Amplification refractory mutation system can be used to identify presence of common mutations in *HBB* gene for diagnosis of β-thalassemia or sickle-cell disease or related hemoglobinopathies.

PCR-RFLP: Polymerase chain reaction followed by restriction fragment length polymorphism can be used for the detection of exon 7 and exon 8 deletion of *SMN1* gene for diagnosis of spinal muscular atrophy.

Multiplex PCR: It can be used to detect hemizygous deletions of exons of the *DMD* gene for diagnosis of Duchenne muscular dystrophy.

Detection of Intron 22 inversion in *F8* gene for diagnosis of hemophilia A can be carried out by long-range PCR or inverse shifting PCR.

Triple primer PCR can be used to diagnose repeat disorders such as Fragile X, Friedreich ataxia, *DMPK* gene-related myotonic dystrophy, spinocerebellar ataxia, Huntington disease, etc.

Quantitative fluorescent PCR (QF-PCR): It can be used to rapidly diagnose common aneuploidies.

Short tandem repeat PCR or variable number of tandem repeat PCR can be used to detect maternal DNA contamination in fetal DNA during prenatal diagnosis.

Congenital infections can be diagnosed by polymerase chain reaction-based tests for toxoplasmosis, cytomegalovirus, rubella, herpes, varicella, etc.

Evidence: Colah et al. (2017) pointed out that ARMS PCR for five or six common mutations is a standard practice to screening for beta thalassemia in the Indian subcontinent. Zeng et al. (2010) pointed out that PCR-RFLP is a standard practice to detect homozygous exon 7 and exon 8 deletions of *SMN1* gene. However, MLPA is a method which has largely replaced PCR-RFLP in many labs. Iskandar et al. (2019) showed that multiplex PCR for 20 exons and muscle promoters of DMD gene can give a diagnostic yield in 44% cases. Deepha et al. (2017) showed that *MLPA* can give a diagnostic yield in 75% patients, of which 92% were deletions and 8% were duplications. Rossetti et al. (2005) invented the inverse PCR method for detection of intron 22 inversion in Hemophilia A which causes 40–45% of severe cases of Hemophilia A. Ciotti et al. (2004) showed that triple primer PCR shows a 100% concordance with Southern blot in molecular diagnosis of Friedreich ataxia. Addis et al. (2012) showed that triple primer PCR is more sensitive than Southern blot in diagnosis of myotonic dystrophy related to *DMPK* gene. Jama et al. (2013) showed that triple primer PCR shows 100% concordance with Southern blot in diagnosis of Huntington disease. Thus, triple primer PCR has replaced Southern blot in molecular diagnosis of repeat disorders. Yamamoto et al. developed a multiplex nested PCR for seven DNA containing pathogens, viz. Toxoplasma, Herpes simplex, varicella zoster virus, parvovirus, cytomegalovirus, adenovirus, and Epstein–Barr virus in

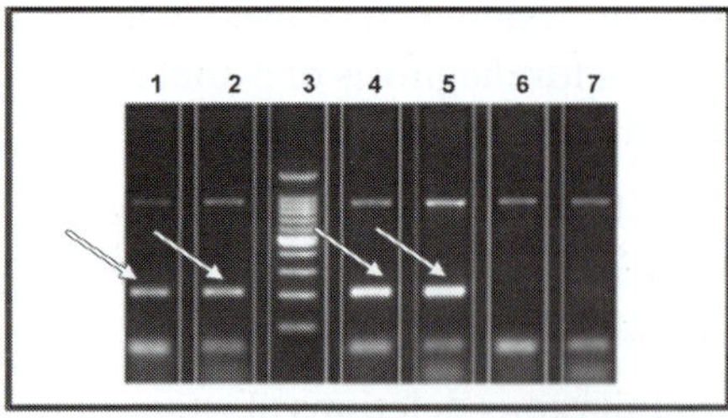

Lane no.		
1	Fetus	Codon 6 A-T mutant allele
2	Fetus	Codon 6 A-T normal allele
3	100 bp molecular weight marker	
4	Positive control	Codon 6 A-T mutant allele
5	Positive control	Codon 6 A-T normal allele
6	Negative control	Codon 6 A-T mutant allele
7	Negative control	Codon 6 A-T normal allele

Results:	The fetus shows the presence of Codon 6 (A-T) mutant allele and Codon 6 (A-T) normal allele, suggesting that the fetus is SICKLE CELL CARRIER.

Fig. 5: Result of ARMS- PCR for prenatal diagnosis of sickle cell disease.

diagnosis of congenital infections. As compared to maternal, fetal, neonatal serology, and placental immunohistochemistry, the PCR method had a 4.6 times higher detection rate.

Limitations: The limitations of PCR are as follows:

- ARMS-PCR has been superseded by *HBB* gene sequencing to reduce false positives or negatives **(Fig. 5)**.
- MLPA tests deletion-duplication analysis has largely replaced multiplex PCR for diagnosis of *MLPA* since it can detect duplications as well as deletions and can also detect heterozygous deletions in carrier individuals, which multiplex PCR cannot.

Q12. What does the term MLPA mean?

Draft recommendations: *MLPA* or multiplex ligation-dependent probe amplification is a genetic technique which uses a set of pairs of probes to detect exon wise deletion duplication (copy number variation) of a gene or detection of methylation-sensitive genomic regions in imprinting disorders.

Q13. What are the applications and limitations of MLPA?

Draft recommendations: The applications of *MLPA* are to diagnose single gene disorders such as Duchenne muscular dystrophy, spinal muscular atrophy, congenital adrenal hyperplasia, and retinoblastoma wherein mutations such as contiguous exonic deletions/duplications are possible or gene conversions are possible due to recombination between gene and pseudogene as in *CYP21A2* gene-related congenital adrenal hyperplasia and Gaucher disease.

It is also used as *MS-MLPA* (methylation-sensitive MLPA) for diagnosis of imprinting disorders such as Prader-Willi syndrome, Angelman syndrome, Beckwith-Wiedemann syndrome, Russell Silver syndrome, etc.

Summary of evidence: Verma et al. (2012) showed the utility of MLPA technique in evaluation of deletion and duplication in Indian patients. They showed an additional diagnostic yield of 5.6% over multiplex PCR. Kaur et al. (2022) showed the utility of MLPA in screening for carriers of *SMN1* gene-related spinal muscular atrophy. They found the carrier frequency of *SMA* to be 1 in 30 individuals. Linh et al. (2023) showed the utility of *MLPA* in diagnosis of *RB1* gene mutations in retinoblastoma patients. They identified deletions in around 12% of their patients. Kim et al. (2022) showed that *MS-MLPA* for Prader-Willi syndrome and Angelman syndrome had a 100% concordance with methylation sensitive PCR.

Limitations: MLPA is not commercially available for several genes.

BIBLIOGRAPHY

1. Addis M, Serrenti M, Meloni C, et al. Triplet-primed PCR is more sensitive than southern blotting-long PCR for the diagnosis of myotonic dystrophy type 1. Genet Test Mol Biomarkers. 2012;16(12):1428-31.
2. Al Arrayed S. Frequency of G6PD deficiency among Bahraini students: a ten years' study. Bah Med Bull. 2010;32(1):18-21.
3. American College of Obstetricians and Gynecologists (ACOG). (2016). Committee Opinion [online] Available from https://www.acog.org/-/media/project/acog/acogorg/clinical/files/committee-opinion/articles/2016/12/microarrays-and-next-generation-sequencing-technology.pdf. [Last accessed November, 2024].
4. Amiel A, Na'amnih W, Tarabeih M. Prenatal Diagnosis and Pregnancy Termination in Jewish and Muslim Women with a Deaf Child in Israel. Children (Basel). 2023;10(9):1438.
5. Ciotti P, Di Maria E, Bellone E, et al. Triplet repeat primed PCR (TP PCR) in molecular diagnostic testing for Friedreich ataxia. J Mol Diagn. 2004;6(4):285-9.
6. Colah R, Italia K, Gorakshakar A. Burden of thalassemia in India: the road map for control. Pediatr Hematol Oncol J [Internet]. 2017;2(4):79-84.
7. Daum H, Peretz T, Laufer N. BRCA mutations and reproduction. Fertil Steril. 2018;109(1):33-8.
8. Deepha S, Vengalil S, Preethish-Kumar V, et al. MLPA identification of dystrophin mutations and in silico evaluation of the predicted protein in dystrophinopathy cases from India. BMC Med Genet. 2017;18(1):67.
9. Donnelly JC, Platt LD, Rebarber A, et al. Association of copy number variants with specific ultrasonographically detected fetal anomalies. Obstet Gynecol. 2014;124(1):83-90.
10. Eggermann K, Bliek J, Brioude F, et al. EMQN best practice guidelines for the molecular genetic testing and reporting of chromosome 11p15 imprinting disorders: Silver-Russell and Beckwith-Wiedemann syndrome. Eur J Hum Genet. 2016;24(10):1377-87.
11. Fu F, Li R, Yu Q, et al. Application of exome sequencing for prenatal diagnosis of fetal structural anomalies: clinical experience and lessons learned from a cohort of 1618 fetuses. Genome Med. 2022;14:123 (2022).
12. Hercher L, Uhlmann WR, Hoffman EP, et al. Prenatal Testing for Adult-Onset Conditions: the Position of the National Society of Genetic Counselors. J Genet Couns. 2016;25(6):1139-45.

13. Iskandar K, Dwianingsih EK, Pratiwi L, et al. The analysis of DMD gene deletions by multiplex PCR in Indonesian DMD/BMD patients: the era of personalized medicine. BMC Res Notes. 2019;12(1):704.
14. Jama M, Millson A, Miller CE, et al. Triplet repeat primed PCR simplifies testing for Huntington disease. J Mol Diagn. 2013;15(2):255-62.
15. Janicki E, De Rademaeker M, Meunier C, et al. Implementation of exome sequencing in prenatal diagnostics: chances and challenges. Diagnostics (Basel). 2023;13(5):860.
16. Kaur A, Kumari A, Kaur A, et al. Carrier frequency of spino-muscular atrophy in individuals of a reproductive age group from North India. J Family Med Prim Care. 2022;11(12):7870-4.
17. Kim B, Park Y, Cho SI, et al. Clinical Utility of Methylation-Specific Multiplex Ligation-Dependent Probe Amplification for the Diagnosis of Prader-Willi Syndrome and Angelman Syndrome. Ann Lab Med. 2022;42(1):79-88.
18. Kujovich JL. Factor V Leiden thrombophilia. Genet Med. 2011;13(1):1-16.
19. Linh DNH, Van Huy N, Nguyen PD, et al. Mutation spectrum of retinoblastoma patients in Vietnam. Mol Genet Genomic Med. 2023;11(11):e2244.
20. Lord J, McMullan DJ, Eberhardt RY, et al. Prenatal Assessment of Genomes and Exomes Consortium. Prenatal exome sequencing analysis in fetal structural anomalies detected by ultrasonography (PAGE): a cohort study. Lancet. 2019; 393(10173):747-57.
21. Manning M, Hudgins L; Professional Practice and Guidelines Committee. Array-based technology and recommendations for utilization in medical genetics practice for detection of chromosomal abnormalities. Genet Med. 2010;12(11):742-5. Erratum in: Genet Med. 2020;22(12):2126.
22. Maya I, Perlman S, Shohat M, et al. Should We Report 15q11.2 BP1-BP2 Deletions and Duplications in the Prenatal Setting? J Clin Med. 2020;9(8):2602.
23. Mellis R, Oprych K, Scotchman E, et al. Diagnostic yield of exome sequencing for prenatal diagnosis of fetal structural anomalies: a systematic review and meta-analysis. Prenat Diagn. 2022;42(6):662-85.
24. Miller DT, Lee K, Abul-Husn NS, et al. Electronic address: documents@ acmg. net. ACMG SF v3.2 list for reporting of secondary findings in clinical exome and genome sequencing: a policy statement of the American College of Medical Genetics and Genomics (ACMG). Genet Med. 2023;25(8): 100866.
25. Richards S, Aziz N, Bale S, et al. Standards and guidelines for the interpretation of sequence variants: a joint consensus recommendation of the American College of Medical Genetics and Genomics and the Association for Molecular Pathology. Genet Med. 2015;17(5):405-24.
26. Rosendahl J, Bödeker H, Mössner J, et al. Hereditary chronic pancreatitis. Orphanet J Rare Dis. 2007;2:1.
27. Rossetti LC, Radic CP, Larripa IB, et al. Genotyping the hemophilia inversion hotspot by use of inverse PCR. Clin Chem. 2005;51(7):1154-8.
28. Sabath DE. Molecular diagnosis of thalassemias and hemoglobinopathies: an aclps critical review. Am J Clin Pathol. 2017;148(1):6-15.
29. Shaffer LG, Agan N, Goldberg JD, et al. American College of Medical Genetics statement of diagnostic testing for uniparental disomy. Genet Med. 2001;3: 206-11.

30. Stuppia L, Antonucci I, Palka G, et al. Use of the MLPA assay in the molecular diagnosis of gene copy number alterations in human genetic diseases. Int J Mol Sci. 2012;13(3):3245-76.
31. Verma PK, Dalal A, Mittal B, et al. Utility of MLPA in mutation analysis and carrier detection for Duchenne muscular dystrophy. Indian J Hum Genet. 2012;18(1):91-4.
32. Wallis JM. Is it ever morally permissible to select for deafness in one's child? Med Health Care Philos. 2020;23(1):3-15.
33. Wang JC, Radcliff J, Coe SJ, et al. Effects of platforms, size filter cutoffs, and targeted regions of cytogenomic microarray on detection of copy number variants and uniparental disomy in prenatal diagnosis: Results from 5026 pregnancies. Prenat Diagn. 2019;39:137-56.
34. Wang M, Cai J, Chen J, et al. PCR Techniques and Their Clinical Applications. IntechOpen. 2024.
35. Wang Y, Yin F, Chai Y, et al. Prenatal diagnosis of fetuses with ultrasound anomalies by whole-exome sequencing in Luoyang city, China. Front Genet. 2024;14:1301439.
36. Wapner RJ, Martin CL, Levy B, et al. Chromosomal microarray versus karyotyping for prenatal diagnosis. N Engl J Med. 2012;367(23):2175-84.
37. Xia M, Yang X, Fu J, et al. Application of chromosome microarray analysis in prenatal diagnosis. BMC Pregnancy Childbirth. 2020;20:696.
38. Yamamoto L, Filho AGA, Queiroz JA, et al. Performance of a multiplex nested polymerase chain reaction in detecting 7 pathogens containing dna in their genomes associated with congenital infections. Arch Pathol Lab Med. 2020;144(1):99-106.
39. Yang Y, Muzny DM, Reid JG, et al. Clinical whole-exome sequencing for the diagnosis of mendelian disorders. N Engl J Med. 2013;369(16):1502-11.
40. Zeng J, Lin Y, Yan A, et al. Establishment of a molecular diagnostic system for spinal muscular atrophy experience from a clinical laboratory in china. J Mol Diagn. 2011;13(1):41-7.

CHAPTER 13

Preimplantation Genetic Testing: Key Questions, Recommendations, and Evidence Review

Keshav Malhotra

Q1. What patients can benefit from "Preimplantation Genetic" testing?

Purpose: The primary goal of Preimplantation Genetic Screening (PGS), now more commonly referred to as Preimplantation Genetic Testing for Aneuploidy (PGT-A), is to identify chromosomal abnormalities in embryos created through IVF before they are transferred to the uterus.

Benefit to patient: By screening embryos for aneuploidy (abnormal numbers of chromosomes), PGT-A aims to improve the chances of a successful pregnancy, reduce the risk of miscarriage, and increase the likelihood of a healthy live birth.

Draft recommendations:

- *Advanced maternal age (AMA):* Recommended for women over 37 years due to the increased risk of aneuploidy.
- *Repeated implantation failure (RIF):* Suggested for identifying chromosomal abnormalities in recurrent unsuccessful implantation cases.
- *Recurrent miscarriage (RM):* May be indicated when there is a known genetic cause; however, it is not routinely recommended without identifiable genetic issues.
- *Severe male factor (SMF):* Could help in selecting viable embryos when male infertility impacts embryo quality.
- *Karyotype analysis:* Especially relevant in cases of chromosomal rearrangements, helping to reduce miscarriage risks.

Summary of evidence:

- *Maternal age:* Women over 37 years have increased risks of aneuploidy and miscarriage, making PGT-A a consideration to improve outcomes (ASRM committee opinion 2017).
- *Repeated implantation failure:* PGT-A can identify chromosomal abnormalities that may contribute to failed implantation attempts, potentially improving the chances of successful pregnancies (ESHRE Guidelines on RPL 2019).
- *Recurrent miscarriage:* PGT-A might be beneficial in certain cases, particularly where genetic causes are known, although guidelines suggest it should not be routinely offered without clear genetic indications (ESHRE Guidelines on RPL 2019).

- *Severe male factor:* PGT-A could help to select viable embryos in cases of severe male infertility, thereby potentially improving the success rates of assisted reproductive technologies (ESHRE Guidelines on RPL 2019).

Research gap:

- *Standardized criteria:* More research is needed to establish clear criteria for the application of PGT-A across different clinical settings, particularly regarding maternal age and history of miscarriages.
- *Long-term outcomes:* Further studies are required to evaluate the long-term health outcomes of children born following PGT-A, particularly concerning the impact of mosaicism and embryo selection criteria.
- *Ethical considerations:* Investigations into the ethical implications of discarding embryos based on genetic testing results, especially regarding the treatment of embryos classified as mosaic or with unclear genetic status.

Q2. Which patients can benefit from PGT-M?

Purpose: Preimplantation Genetic Testing for Monogenic Disorders (PGT-M) enables couples at risk of passing on specific genetic disorders to have children free from those conditions by screening embryos before implantation.

Benefit to patients: This testing is especially valuable for families with a history of severe genetic diseases, such as cystic fibrosis, Tay-Sachs disease, or Huntington's disease, as it allows for the selection of embryos without the targeted disorder. PGT-M provides couples with increased control over their reproductive choices, minimizing the emotional and financial strain of caring for a child with a debilitating condition. It also offers significant practical benefits, including reducing the risk of miscarriage associated with certain genetic abnormalities and avoiding the need for invasive prenatal testing and the potential for difficult pregnancy-related decisions. By reducing genetic risks, PGT-M improves the likelihood of a healthy pregnancy and a better quality of life for the child, empowering patients to make informed, values-driven choices about family planning.

Draft recommendations:

- *Pathogenic/likely pathogenic variants:* Recommended for pathogenic germline genetic variants with significant health impacts, manifesting at birth, in childhood, or adulthood. Additional studies (functional or family-based) may be necessary to confirm the clinical relevance of certain variants.
- *Carrier status:* If a pathogenic variant is identified in both the proband and one parent, PGT-M is suggested, especially when a single gene is implicated, and haplotypes associated with the disorder are well-characterized within the family.

- *Testing in absence of pathogenic variant:* For families with a clear history of X-linked recessive disorders but no identified variant in the proband, PGT-M can be offered if family history supports haplotype-based risk assessment.
- *Exclusions: Variants of unknown significance (VUS)*—PGT-M is not recommended for variants lacking predictive information about the phenotype.
- *Uncertain genetic diagnoses:* Testing is avoided when genetic/molecular heterogeneity or inheritance patterns are unclear.

Summary of evidence:

- *Historical context:* Originally intended to prevent severe childhood-onset conditions, PGT-M's scope now includes a broader range of genetic disorders, including those with mild or variable phenotypes, later onset, and lower penetrance. A survey by Harper et al. (2021) found strong support among genetic counselors for PGT-M in conditions with lower penetrance, citing patient autonomy.
- *Guideline limitations:* Currently, formal guidelines on PGT-M applications are limited, with ethical and clinical factors varying across institutions. Establishing transparent internal policies is recommended to guide patient decisions. Several institutions have developed policies to guide PGT-M practices for a range of genetic conditions, aiming for consistency in patient's counseling (ESHRE, 2020).

Research gaps:

- *Patient's use:* Unclear data on how many couples proceed with PGT-M after initial consultation, suggesting potential barriers to access.
- *Patient's motivations:* Limited quantitative data on motivations, satisfaction, and decision-making of patients consulting for PGT-M.
- *Reference materials:* A lack of reliable pedigree-based and genomic reference materials affects PGT-M accuracy and efficiency, especially given the technical challenges of testing single cells.
- *Patient's knowledge:* A significant portion (40–80%) of patients report not receiving sufficient information about PGT-M.

Q3. What are the requirements for laboratory standards and equipment in performing PGT?

Overview: Performing Preimplantation Genetic Testing (PGT) requires rigorous laboratory standards and specialized equipment to ensure accuracy, reliability, and patient's safety. Key requirements include a dedicated, contamination-free area for embryo biopsies, clinical-grade equipment calibrated to handle single-cell analysis, and stringent protocols for maintaining sterility. Essential equipment includes an inverted microscope with laser-assisted hatching capabilities, precise micromanipulators, and a constant power supply to ensure uninterrupted procedures. Additionally, laboratory environments must meet regulated standards for air quality, positive pressure, and temperature control to protect embryo viability. These strict standards directly benefit patients by enhancing the accuracy of genetic testing, reducing the risk of contamination, and preserving embryo integrity, ultimately increasing the likelihood of successful outcomes. Such meticulous care in the PGT process gives patients' confidence in the results, supports informed reproductive choices, and improves their chances of having a healthy child.

Draft recommendations:

Laboratory infrastructure:

- *Dedicated biopsy areas:* Perform oocyte and embryo biopsies in specially designated laboratory areas designed for single or few-cell processing. Use physical isolation to prevent contamination, with measures to detect contamination actively in place.
- *Licensing and compliance:* Obtain appropriate licensing for biopsy and genetic testing procedures according to local regulatory requirements.

Equipment:

- *Clinical-grade equipment:* Use clinical-grade equipment specifically designed for PGT procedures. Maintain regular calibration and servicing schedules and follow standardized operating procedures (SOPs).
- *Uninterrupted power supply (UPS):* Equip critical laboratory devices with a UPS to maintain consistent power during procedures.
- *Work surface and equipment sterilization:* Decontaminate work surfaces and equipment using DNA-specific decontamination solutions or bleach; avoid using 70% ethanol. In preamplification steps, avoid automated pipetting systems and multichannel pipettes to minimize contamination risk.
- *Optional multichannel pipettes/automation:* While multichannel pipettes and automated systems can reduce mislabeling risks post-amplification, they are best reserved for downstream processes.

Summary of evidence: The infrastructure and equipment in an embryology laboratory, particularly in high-volume IVF settings, should include areas designed specifically for PGT biopsies. In high-demand settings, a separate biopsy room can improve workflow, maintaining quality air standards, positive pressure, and access controls. According to the "Revised Guidelines for Good Practice in IVF Laboratories," adherence to environmental standards and safety protocols helps protect biological materials from contamination. Studies underscore that dedicated biopsy areas enhance workflow and reduce contamination risks, which are critical for successful PGT outcomes. Compliance with local health and laboratory safety regulations has been associated with improved laboratory practices and adherence to safety standards. Ensuring precision and calibration in equipment reduces variability in biopsy outcomes, essential for reliable genetic analysis. Backup power sources protect valuable biological samples from damage due to power fluctuations, supporting consistent laboratory function. Using DNA-specific cleaning solutions has been shown to reduce cross-contamination risks, ensuring sample integrity. Automation postamplification minimizes human error without compromising early-stage sample integrity (ESHRE PGT Consortium, 2020).

Research gaps:

- *Laboratory infrastructure and environment:* More data are needed to determine the optimal laboratory conditions (e.g., air quality, temperature, and positive pressure) that guarantee contamination-free embryo handling and biopsy procedures. Research could clarify whether separate biopsy rooms offer distinct advantages over designated spaces within IVF labs, particularly regarding contamination control.
- *Microscope and equipment standards:* Specific evidence-backed standards for magnification, laser types, and micromanipulator configurations could improve biopsy accuracy and support embryo viability in PGT laboratories. Standardizing equipment configurations could lead to more consistent PGT outcomes and improve reliability in different laboratory settings.

Q4. How to handle reagents, samples, and prevent contamination in PGT laboratories?

Overview: In Preimplantation Genetic Testing (PGT) laboratories, handling reagents and samples with precision and care is essential to maintain sample integrity and prevent contamination.

Draft recommendations:

- *Use of protective gear:* Full protective clothing should be worn for DNA amplification processes involving single or few cells. This includes:
  - Clean and nonsterile surgical gowns (changed regularly)
  - Hair covers, face masks covering both nose and mouth, and shoe covers or dedicated laboratories shoes
  - Well-fitting gloves (preferably nitrile, not vinyl), changed frequently.
- *Specialized clothing in IVF centers:* Use low particle-shedding protective clothing, nonpowdered gloves, and surgical masks to further reduce particulate and DNA contamination.
- *Storage in designated areas:* Store preamplification materials and reagents separately from DNA sources, ideally in a dedicated preamplification area.

- *Ready-to-use reagents and plasticware:* Use ready-to-use, molecular biology-grade reagents and DNA-free, DNase-free plastic-ware, including filter tips. Validate all reagents for their purity and efficacy.
- *Batch number recording:* Record batch or lot numbers for reagents to ensure traceability as part of laboratory quality standards.
- *Reagent decontamination:* Decontaminate reagents using UV-C irradiation or autoclaving in a dedicated PGT autoclave if reagents are prepared in-house.
- *Temperature and handling precautions:* Store reagents at recommended temperatures, avoid rapid temperature changes, and refrain from vortexing sensitive reagents.
- *Avoid contact with tube openings:* Minimize contamination risks by avoiding contact with the inside or lid of reaction tubes with gloved hands, and change gloves if contact occurs. Change pipette tips immediately if they touch the tube cap or outside of tubes.

Summary of evidence: To prevent DNA contamination in PGT laboratories, it is recommended to follow stringent protocols for surface and equipment decontamination. Cleaning work surfaces with DNA-specific solutions or 10% bleach before procedures has been shown effective; however, bleach is less ideal for use within the embryology lab due to its reactive nature. Alternatives, such as DNA decontamination solutions, are preferred over 70% ethanol, which does not fully eliminate DNA residues. Studies show that dedicated protective gear reduces contamination risk, especially in preamplification processes where single cells are highly susceptible to contamination from external DNA sources. Low-shedding protective clothing significantly reduces airborne particles, which is critical in IVF and PGT laboratories to maintain sample purity. Separate storage has been shown to reduce cross-contamination between DNA samples and reagents. Ready-to-use and molecular-grade reagents reduce variability in results and ensure high-quality outcomes for PGT. Consistent reagent tracking and limited handling have been shown to improve reproducibility and reduce cross-contamination risks. Maintaining stable storage conditions help to prevent degradation of sensitive reagents and ensures consistency in DNA amplification results (European Society of Human Reproduction and Embryology, 2020). Careful handling of reaction tubes and pipette tips has been shown to significantly reduce contamination, essential for accurate PGT results.

Research gaps:

Decontamination protocols: Clear and standardized protocols for DNA contamination prevention are lacking, particularly regarding handling single cells or small cell quantities. Future research should assess the comparative efficacy of bleach, DNA decontamination solutions, and traditional cleaning agents like ethanol for different lab environments. While bleach and DNA-specific cleaners are commonly used, further studies are needed to establish best practices that ensure complete DNA decontamination without compromising embryo viability in PGT settings.

Q5. What are the preclinical workup requirements for a PGT case?

Overview: A comprehensive preclinical workup for PGT should ensure complete administrative, patient, and genetic information, allowing accurate interpretation and application of the PGT results.

Draft recommendations:

- *Report identification:* Each report should have a title, a unique identifier for document control, and pagination with patient identifiers on every page.
- *Contact details:* The report should include the date, referring physician's name and address, and contact information for the IVF/PGT center.
- *Diagnostician information:* Identification and signature of the diagnostician(s) involved should be included.
- *Patient's information:* Full name or a unique code, date of birth, and gender of the patient(s) should be recorded to ensure clear patient identification.
- *Sample information:* Dates for DNA sample collection and arrival should be noted.
- *Genetic information of family members:* Include family genetic information where possible and ensure compliance with GDPR/local privacy laws.
- *PGT-SR outcomes:* For PGT-SR cases, include an overview of likely segregation patterns to inform on potential outcomes.
- *Testing information:* Specify clinical indications, testing type, and parental karyotypes.
- *Genetic tests used:* Indicate specific genetic tests, methods, software, and commercial kits (include references and versions used).
- *Result reporting:* The report should provide a clear interpretation and summary of results, highlighting any error rates, limitations, and misdiagnosis risks.
- *Assumptions in haplotyping:* For reports based on haplotyping, include assumptions regarding sample identity and family relationships.
- *Protocol communication:* Details on the biopsy type, number of cells used, and any associated specifics should be communicated to the patient and the IVF center.
- *Prenatal testing options:* When a pregnancy results from PGT, remind parents about residual misdiagnosis risks and available prenatal testing options. IVF centers should aim to follow up with parents on prenatal or postnatal results.

- *Sample retention:* Adhere to local guidelines for sample and record storage. Where guidelines are absent, store FISH slides, DNA products, or other materials for a minimum of one year for transferred or frozen embryos. Consider extended storage based on embryo cryopreservation duration and birth outcomes.

Summary of evidence: PGT clinical reports require secure and clear reporting of findings, including cycle-specific details, dates, biopsy information, and testing methods. Accurate administrative details reduce errors and improve traceability, ensuring secure and compliant handling of PGT records. Accurate patient information is essential to avoid misidentification, which can impact treatment outcomes. Clear genetic records help to determine inheritance patterns, essential for accurate PGT diagnosis. Detailing testing methods and equipment improves result reliability and quality control in the PGT process. Clear result summaries and risk disclosures are essential for patient comprehension and decision-making. Following up on prenatal testing enhances patient understanding of residual risks and promotes informed decision-making. Longer storage periods for samples and records allow for retrospective analyses, supporting patient's follow-up and quality assurance.

Research gaps: Limited evidence on optimal reporting formats suggests a need for standardized formats to improve communication with IVF centers and patient understanding.

- *Standardized report formats:* Limited research on report formats creates a risk of misinterpretation by IVF centers and patients. Studies should evaluate which formats maximize clarity and comprehension.
- *Prenatal follow-up protocols:* Insufficient guidelines exist for patient education and follow-up communication. Future studies could investigate the impact of different follow-up protocols on patient's outcomes and satisfaction.

Q6. Is this treatment add-on safe?

Overview: Preimplantation Genetic Testing (PGT) is generally considered safe, especially when performed in established laboratories by trained professionals. While PGT is a low-risk procedure, there are some considerations. There is a very small chance of embryo damage during the biopsy, though advancements in biopsy techniques and equipment have reduced this risk significantly.

Draft recommendations:

- *No additional risk to patient:* Preimplantation Genetic Testing for Aneuploidy (PGT-A) does not increase health risks to the individual undergoing treatment; rather, it involves embryo biopsy, which can pose limited risks primarily to the embryo itself.

- *Accuracy limitations:* While PGT-A technologies like Next-Generation Sequencing (NGS) are generally accurate, error rates persist. Factors such as biopsy timing, technical sensitivity, and mosaicism can lead to diagnostic inaccuracies. Studies show that both false-positive and false-negative results can occur, potentially leading to the misidentification of chromosomal abnormalities.
- *Impact on embryo selection:* Misdiagnosis could result in the discard of potentially healthy embryos, thereby reducing the number of embryos available for transfer. Research by Mastenbroek S et al. (2011) highlights instances where PGT-A results led to the unnecessary discard of embryos, affecting overall pregnancy chances.
- *Mosaic embryos:* Mosaic embryos—those with both normal and abnormal cells—are sometimes discarded even though they can lead to healthy pregnancies. Studies indicate that while mosaic embryos may have lower implantation rates compared to euploid embryos, they can still produce healthy live births (Fragouli et al., 2019).
- *Chromosomal abnormalities:* In cases where all embryos are found to be aneuploid, none may be available for transfer, thus reducing the likelihood of pregnancy. PGT-A has shown the potential to reduce miscarriage rates, but it does not guarantee pregnancy success (Gleicher et al., 2021).
- *Potential embryo damage:* The biopsy process used to obtain cells from the embryo can occasionally cause minor morphological damage, potentially impacting developmental viability. Most embryos withstand cell removal well, though some may experience slight damage that could influence implantation success.

Summary of evidence:

- *Procedural safety for the patient:* Studies have shown that PGT-A does not introduce risks to the individual undergoing IVF since it is primarily a biopsy of the embryo rather than an invasive procedure for the patient.
- *Diagnostic accuracy concerns:* Even with advanced techniques like NGS, factors like biopsy quality, timing, and mosaicism can lead to misdiagnosis. Greco et al. (2015) identified that despite advancements, false-positive and false-negative results are still a concern, affecting embryo viability assessments.
- *Embryo selection impact:* The accuracy limitations of PGT-A can result in the discard of viable embryos. Mastenbroek S et al. (2011) demonstrated that diagnostic errors in PGT-A could reduce the embryo pool, potentially lowering success rates.
- *Mosaic embryo viability:* Fragouli et al. (2019) discussed that mosaic embryos can lead to healthy pregnancies, though they are generally discarded in some clinics due to their lower implantation rates.

- *Embryo biopsy risks:* While biopsy can minimally impact embryo morphology, most embryos continue to develop post-biopsy, though minor risks persist.

Research gaps:

- *Misdiagnosis rates and risk of false results:* Treff et al. (2021) highlighted that misdiagnosis persists, with approximately 5–10% of embryos labeled as mosaic still potentially leading to live births, underscoring the difficulty of assessing viability solely based on PGT-A.
- *Mosaicism interpretation:* A lack of consensus exists on the clinical significance of mosaic embryos. Greco et al. (2015) observed that some mosaic embryos result in healthy births, though certain degrees of mosaicism correlate with lower implantation rates.
- *Impact on specific patient populations:* PGT-A's effectiveness in improving live birth rates is mixed, especially among younger women. PGT-A may not significantly benefit younger women with good prognosis, raising questions about which patient groups benefit most.
- *Laboratory practice standardization:* Variations in laboratory practices can significantly affect PGT-A results, calling for standardized guidelines to enhance reproducibility and reliability.
- *Ethical considerations of mosaic embryo disposal:* Orvieto et al. (2017) discussed ethical concerns, emphasizing that some mosaic embryos may still lead to healthy pregnancies, creating ethical dilemmas for clinicians and patients.
- *Cost-effectiveness:* Cost-effectiveness analysis found that while PGT-A may benefit specific patient populations, it may not be cost-effective across all patient groups.

BIBLIOGRAPHY

1. Cimadomo D, Capalbo A, Ubaldi FM, et al. The impact of biopsy on human embryo developmental potential during preimplantation genetic diagnosis. Biomed Res Int. 2016;2016:7193075.
2. ESHRE Guideline Group on RPL. ESHRE guideline: recurrent pregnancy loss. Hum Reprod Open. 2019;1:hoy004.
3. ESHRE PGT Consortium. (2019). Data Collection and Reporting Standards in PGT: ESHRE PGT Consortium Online Database. [online] Available from https://eshre.eu. [Last accessed November, 2024].
4. ESHRE PGT Consortium. Guidelines for PGT laboratories: Contamination prevention, infrastructure, and equipment standards. Hum Reprod. 2020;35(5):1012-20.
5. ESHRE PGT Consortium. The current state of preimplantation genetic testing for monogenic disorders (PGT-M): Guidelines and practices. Fertil Steril. 2020;114(2):304-12.

6. European Society of Human Reproduction and Embryology (ESHRE). (2021). Guidelines on Follow-Up Communication and Risk Counseling in PGT. ESHRE. [online] Available from https://eshre.eu. [Last accessed November, 2024].
7. European Society of Human Reproduction and Embryology (ESHRE). Revised guidelines for PGT laboratory procedures. Hum Reprod. 2020;35(9):1205-15.
8. Fragouli E, Munne S, Wells D. The cytogenetic constitution of human blastocysts: insights from comprehensive chromosome screening strategies. Hum Reprod Update. 2019;25(1):15-33.
9. Gleicher N, Patrizio P, Brivanlou A. Preimplantation genetic testing for aneuploidy–a castle built on sand. Trends Mol Med. 2021;27(8):731-42.
10. Greco E, et al. Preimplantation genetic diagnosis for aneuploidy screening in advanced maternal age." N Engl J Med. 2015.
11. Harper J. PGT equipment and biopsy area specifications: recommendations for best practices. J Reprod Biotechnol. 2021;12(3):287-95.
12. Mastenbroek S, Twisk M, van der Veen F, et al. Preimplantation genetic screening: a systematic review and meta-analysis of RCTs. Hum Reprod Update. 2011;17(4):454-66.
13. Orvieto R, et al. Ethics of mosaic embryo discard in PGT-A. Reprod Biomed Online. 2017.
14. Practice Committee of the American Society for Reproductive Medicine. Aging and infertility: a committee opinion. Fertil Steril. 2017;107(3):591-600.
15. Smith A, Jones R, Patel N. Administrative requirements in genetic reporting for reproductive medicine. J Assist Reprod Genet. 2022;39(2):211-23.
16. Treff NR, Marin D. The "mosaic" embryo: misconceptions and misinterpretations in preimplantation genetic testing for aneuploidy. Fertil Steril. 2021; 116(5): 1205-11.

CHAPTER 14

Cancer Genetics for Women

Rajiv Sarin

Q1. When to suspect a cancer is inherited and when is genetic testing indicated?

Draft recommendations: Inherited predisposition should be suspected in patients with personal and significant family history of same or related types of cancer especially when it is early onset, bilateral or multiple primary cancer; physical phenotypic features or specific histological or molecular features suggestive of underlying gene mutation. These individuals should be offered genetic counseling and appropriate germline genetic testing.

Background and evidence: Traditionally, a cancer was considered to be hereditary and genetic testing was advised only if there was significant family history of same or related types of cancers or a classical syndromic phenotype. With widespread germline testing using multigene NGS it is recognized that a significant proportion of individuals with a germline mutation in a high penetrance gene such as *BRCA1* or *BRCA2* or *MLH1* gene have little or no family history or the classical syndromic presentation of Hereditary Breast Ovarian Cancer (HBOC) Syndrome or Lynch Syndrome. This is because of variable penetrance of mutation in different genes and the differences in penetrance of genes like *BRCA1* and *BRCA2* between males and females with fathers often being asymptomatic carriers. Genetic testing options are provided to individuals in whom there is a reasonable prospect of finding a pathogenic or likely pathogenic germline mutation in a moderate to high penetrance gene which could help guide their cancer prevention, tailored treatment and extended family testing.

While a significant family history of cancer continues to be the most definitive indication for genetic testing, even in absence of family history, a cancer is suspected to be of possible hereditary nature and genetic testing is recommended to rule out germline mutation if:

- A person develops cancer at an age unusually young for that cancer, e.g., breast, or colorectal cancer <40 years or ovarian or endometrial cancer <50 years of age.
- A person develops cancer in paired organs, such as both breasts, kidneys, or eyes.
- A person develops more than one primary cancer, such as ovarian cancer and breast cancer or colon and endometrium.

- Phenotypic features of specific hereditary syndromes, e.g., polyps, skin patches, etc.
- Pathology or IHC or other tests on the tumor suggests it to be of genetic type, e.g.:
  - Triple negative breast cancer—TNBC (ER, PR, and Her2 are negative.)
  - Ovarian cancer which is high grade and epithelial carcinoma
  - Endometrial or colorectal cancer which has Microsatellite Instability (MSI High) or MMR deficient (dMMR)
  - Some rare tumors, e.g., male breast cancer, choroid plexus carcinoma, etc.
- Patients with metastatic cancer with at least 5% possibility of finding a germline mutation in a gene based on which targeted therapy may be offered, e.g., *BRCA* or *MMR*
- Somatic tumor NGS testing identifies in a gene relevant for hereditary cancer, a mutation at a high variant allele frequency (VAF), suggesting its possible germline origin.

This clinicopathological context and indication for germline genetic testing is now universally included in the clinical practice guidelines from all major professional bodies in North America and Europe. These include the US National Cancer Centres Network (NCCN), American and European Society of Medical Oncology (ASCO and ESMO) guidelines and the Indian National Cancer Grid Guidelines.

Gaps in knowledge: The north American guidelines from ASCO and NCCN that are adopted globally are progressively relaxing the criteria for germline genetic testing. Thus, the age cut-off for sporadic TNBC has been removed, sporadic non-TNBC breast cancer age has been relaxed from 50 years to 65 years and all nonmucinous epithelial ovarian cancers, and all high risk or metastatic prostate cancers are advised germline genetic testing. The recommendation of panels of genes has also increased from only *BRCA1, BRCA2* to multigene panels including mismatch repair (MMR) and several other genes. However, there is little information on the incremental yield of relaxing the testing criteria or the additional genes in the NGS panel in different populations. This is particularly relevant for the Indian population with limited access to genetic counselling and testing, scantly population level data and higher rates of variants of uncertain clinical significance (VUS). Germline mutations in genes other than *BRCA1/BRCA2* are seen in 25% breast cancer cases and in 15% ovarian cancer cases (Tata Hospital Registry). However, to detect mutation in these additional genes there is a corresponding increase in the VUS rates.

Q2. What is the burden of inherited cancers in Indian women and how to bridge the care gap?

Draft recommendations: There is an unrecognized burden of inherited cancers in Indian women with approximately 100,000 individuals in 25,000 families each year. However, there are very limited cancer genetic services to cater to these families who need genetic counselling, adequate and timely genetic testing, cancer screening, prevention and therapeutic advice based on the genetic test results. Mainstreaming of genetic testing by the practising oncologists and gynecologists is a pragmatic approach recently developed in Europe. Patients without significant family history or psychosocial issues are sent directly for genetic testing by their physician and if a germline mutation or VUS is identified they are then referred to the specialized Cancer Genetics Clinic (CGC) for detailed counselling advice and family member testing. This reduces time and resources as compared to the conventional model of sending all patients first for pretest counselling to the CGC, then genetic testing and then posttest counseling at the CGC before the patient returns to their oncologists.

Background and evidence: As per the recent WHO GLOBOCAN data for 2022, each year 722,000 women in India are diagnosed with cancer. Breast cancer is the most common cancer (192,000 cases) in Indian women followed by cancer of cervix (127,000 cases), ovary (47,000 cases), oral (36,000 cases), and endometrium (17,000 cases). The proportion of the common cancers that are inherited due to a germline mutation vary from as high as 20% for ovarian cancer, 5–10% for breast and endometrial cancer and 1–2% for cervical cancer or oral cancer. Thus, each year there are approximately 25,000 new breast or gynecological cancers due to inherited predisposition. The index cases and their families need genetic counseling, genetic testing, high-risk screening and prevention as well as precision medicine with targeted therapy (e.g., PARP inhibitors for germline or somatic mutations in *BRCA1/2*) or immunotherapy (e.g., germline mutation in *MMR* genes or *MMR*-deficient tumors). However, there are very few trained cancer genetic counselors, cancer geneticists, or specialized cancer genetics clinics in India. The Cancer Genetics Clinic running for over two decades at the Tata Memorial Hospital Mumbai registers 2,500 new families every year. However, most states and even metropolitan cities in India and other Asian countries are underserved with no specialized cancer genetics clinics or services. Moreover, the guidelines-based indications for germline genetic testing are being continuously expanded for common cancers like, breast, ovary, prostate, colorectal and endometrial cancers.

The barriers in providing cancer genetic services are not limited to lack of resources. There is a need to develop infrastructure and human resources, establish hub and spoke referral network, and generate India specific data through collaborative research and data sharing. These aspects are not unique to India and most Asian and other developing countries face a similar situation. Even in western countries genetic counseling has become a bottleneck due to sudden increase in the indications for cancer genetic testing such as all epithelial ovarian cancers and many more breast and prostate cancer cases requiring testing.

Gaps in knowledge: Mainstreaming of genetic testing by practicing oncologists and gynecologists that helped to tide over this surge of genetic testing in the west has also been pilot tested in some Asian countries. However, its applicability in India and other developing countries may require modifications to account for the major differences in the literacy and awareness level of the patients and continued medical education systems lacking in the field of cancer genetics. A mainstreaming programe being developed at the Tata Memorial Hospital is taking into account the sociocultural differences in the patient population and the Indian health care set up. This needs to be evaluated for its implementation at other Indian centers. A PG diploma in Cancer Genetics and Counseling has been started to fill the gap of Cancer Genetic Counselors across the country.

Q3. If a germline variant of uncertain clinical significance (VUS) is identified, should it be a part of the genetic test report and considered in the counseling process?

Draft recommendations: A VUS in a gene related to the disease condition being evaluated should be included in the genetic test report and the associated uncertainty should be explained in the genetic counseling process—why the rare variant has been called a VUS and that it cannot be used for advising cancer screening, prevention, targeted therapy or testing in the family. They should be advised what additional information can be gathered to reclassify the VUS such as IHC for MMR gene or other functional assays or checking whether or not the same variant is found in the cancer affected members of the family (co-segregation). It should be emphasized that the family should contact the testing laboratory if in future their personal or family history changes and annually to know if the variant has been reclassified as likely benign (of no concern) or likely pathogenic (requiring specific cancer screening and prevention).

Background and evidence: Currently, the American College of Medical Genetics (ACMG) 5-tier variant classification system uses several criteria to classify any germline variant as disease causing Pathogenic (tier 5) or Likely Pathogenic (tier 4) or not causing the related hereditary condition—Likely Benign (tier 2) or Benign (tier 1). If scientific and genomic databases and scientific literature is unable to confidently classify a rare gene variant to cause or not cause the related hereditary condition, it is called a VUS (tier 3). No definitive recommendations can be made for screening, prevention or therapy of the tested individual or family for the VUS. Based on personal or family history, age and sex, their physicians may recommend specific cancer screening or suggest for or against a treatment approach. The ambiguous nature of the results can sometimes lead to misinterpretation of results by the tested person, family and sometimes their doctors. Hence, a post-test genetic counseling is essential for these issues to be understood and any doubts clarified.

Gaps in knowledge: In absence of reliable information on the frequency and zygosity of a variant in the healthy population it becomes difficult to classify a variant. As a result, when compared to the well-characterized Caucasian populations, VUS rates are higher in other populations including south Asians. Healthy individuals from these ethnic groups are poorly represented in population genomic databases. There is a need to generate population level genomic data and deposit them in databases used for variant classification. Attempts to reclassify a VUS do not change its classification, i.e., remains as VUS in 50–60% cases, 40% are reclassified as Likely benign and 5–10% are reclassified as Likely Pathogenic with clinical implications. Strengthening of variant reclassification programs and depositing Indian data in the genomic population databases (gnomAD or 1000 Genome) and disease databases (ClinVar) can greatly reduce the VUS rates.

Q4. What are the cancer risks in women with germline mutations in *BRCA1, BRCA2,* and contentious issues in genetic counseling?

Draft recommendations: Women with a germline pathogenic variant (mutations) in *BRCA1* or *BRCA2* gene have a very high lifetime risk for cancer. The breast cancer risk is 70–80% with the risk starting in early 20s and the ovarian cancer risk is 30–40% with the risk starting in mid 30s. These women need genetic counseling about their cancer risks and their options for screening, chemoprevention, risk reducing surgery, and targeted therapy if they develop advanced cancer. There is greater uncertainty about cancer risks, screening, prevention, and targeted therapy for mutation in other related genes with intermediate or uncertain penetrance.

Background and evidence: Since the identification of *BRCA1* gene in 1994 and *BRCA2* gene in 1995, a large body of literature has emerged.

Breast and Ovarian cancer risk in female carriers of *BRCA1, BRCA2,* or related genes

- *Breast Cancer (risk starting from early 20s and 30–50% cases having bilateral cancer)*
    - *BRCA1:* 70–80% (usually Triple Negative)
    - *BRCA2:* 60–70% (usually ER +ve)
    - *TP53:* 70–80% (usually Her2 +ve)
    - *PALB2:* 50%
    - *CDH1:* 50% (usually Lobular carcinoma)
    - *ATM, CHEK2, RAD51C/D,* etc.: 20–40%
- *Screening and Prevention for Breast Cancer risk:*
    - Monthly breast self-examination: 6-monthly clinical breast examination and annual breast MRI alternating with mammograms after the age of 30 years (if breast is not dense).

- Detailed counseling about the OPTION of Prophylactic Bilateral Nipple and skin sparing Mastectomy with reconstruction; extent of risk reduction and procedure associated complications.
- Chemoprevention using tamoxifen can reduce the risk of *BRCA2* associated breast cancer by 50% but not for *BRCA1* associated breast cancer which are usually ER/PR negative.

- *Ovary cancer (risk starting from mid-30s and majority are high-grade serous adenocarcinoma)*
    - *BRCA1:* 40%
    - *BRCA2:* 30–40%
    - *PALB2, ATM, RAD51D,* etc.: 5–15%
- *Screening and prevention for ovary cancer risk:* Ovarian cancer screening with transvaginal ultrasound or serum *CA125* has limitations in detecting early stage of ovarian cancer. Hence, risk reducing salpingo-oophorectomy (RRSO) with or without hysterectomy is strongly recommended after completion of family at age of 35 years for *BRCA1* and age of 40 years for *BRCA2* mutations. For genes such as *ATM, CHEK2, RAD51,* and a few others with ovarian cancer risk of 5–10%, RRSO may or may not be considered at or after the age of 40 years. A stronger recommendation of RRSO in carriers of these intermediate penetrance genes can be made if they have a family history of ovarian cancer.
- *Therapeutic implications of germline or somatic mutation in BRCA and other HRR genes:* Double-strand DNA damage is repaired mainly by the homologous recombination repair (HRR) pathway. HRR pathway is defective if there is a loss of function mutation (germline or tumor) in one of the *HRR* genes like *BRCA, ATM, PALB2,* etc. Several randomized trials, including a recent meta-analysis has shown survival benefit with the use of PARP inhibitors in breast cancer and ovarian cancer patients with germline or somatic *BRCA1/2* mutation.

Gaps in knowledge: While much is known about the age and sex specific risks for different cancers for the *BRCA1* and *BRCA2* genes, the data is uncertain about intermediate penetrance genes such as *CHEK2, ATM, RAD51,* etc. Even for the high penetrance *BRCA1* and *BRCA2* genes, the cumulative risk or penetrance in the Asian and Indian population is not well known.

BIBLIOGRAPHY

1. Bedrosian I, Somerfield MR, Achatz MI, et al. Germline Testing in Patients With Breast Cancer: ASCO-Society of Surgical Oncology Guideline. J Clin Oncol. 2024;42(5):584-604.
2. Bray F, Laversanne M, Sung H, et al. Global cancer statistics 2022: GLOBOCAN estimates of incidence and mortality worldwide for 36 cancers in 185 countries. CA Cancer J Clin. 2024;74(3):229-63.

3. Chang J, Seng S, Yoo J, et al. Clinical management of patients at risk for hereditary breast cancer with variants of uncertain significance in the era of multigene panel testing. Ann Surg Oncol. 2019;26(10):3389-96.
4. Daly MB, Pal T, Berry MP, et al. Genetic/familial high-risk assessment: breast, ovarian, and pancreatic, version 2.2021, NCCN clinical practice guidelines in oncology. J Nat Comprehen Cancer Netw. 2021;19(1):77-102.
5. George A, Riddell D, Seal S, et al. Implementing rapid, robust, cost-effective, patient-centred, routine genetic testing in ovarian cancer patients. Sci Rep. 2016;6:29506.
6. Gulia S, Kannan S, Ghosh J, et al. Maintenance therapy with a poly (ADP-ribose) polymerase inhibitor in patients with newly diagnosed advanced epithelial ovarian cancer: individual patient data and trial-level meta-analysis. ESMO Open. 2022;7(5):100558.
7. Nakamura S, Kwong A, Kim SW, et al. Current Status of the Management of Hereditary Breast and Ovarian Cancer in Asia: First report by the Asian BRCA Consortium. Public Health Genomics. 2016;19(1):53-60.
8. National Cancer Grid. (2024). NCG Guidelines. [online] Available from https://www.ncgindia.org/cancer-guidelines. [Last accessed Nov., 2024].
9. Sarin R. Cancer Genetics. In: Kamath SA (Ed). API Textbook of Medicine, 11th Edition. New Delhi: Jaypee Brothers Medical Publishers (P) Ltd.; 2019.
10. Sun X, Wang X, Zhang J, et al. Efficacy and safety of PARP inhibitors in patients with BRCA-mutated advanced breast cancer: a meta-analysis and systematic review. Breast. 2021;60:26-34.
11. Tung N, Ricker C, Messersmith H, et al. Selection of Germline Genetic Testing Panels in Patients With Cancer: ASCO Guideline. JCO. 2024;42:2599-615.
12. Tung NM, Boughey JC, Pierce LJ, et al. Management of Hereditary Breast Cancer: American Society of Clinical Oncology, American Society for Radiation Oncology, and Society of Surgical Oncology Guideline. J Clin Oncol. 2020;38:2080-106.
13. Tutt ANJ, Garber JE, Kaufman B, et al.; OlympiA Clinical Trial Steering Committee and Investigators. Adjuvant Olaparib for Patients with BRCA1 or BRCA2-Mutated Breast Cancer. N Engl J Med. 2021;384:2394-405.
14. Walsh N, Cooper A, Dockery A, et al. Variant reclassification and clinical implications. J Med Genet. 2024;61:207-21.
15. Yoon SY, Wong SW, Lim J, et al. Oncologist-led BRCA counselling improves access to cancer genetic testing in middle income Asian country with no significant impact on psychosocial outcomes. J Med Genet. 2022;59(3):220-9.

15

CHAPTER

Research Advances and Future Directions in Obstetric Genetics

Usha Dave, Pratiksha Chheda

Q1. What is the role of genomics in NIPS and prenatal diagnosis?

Noninvasive prenatal screening (NIPS) has transformed the landscape of prenatal testing, enabling the detection of a wide range of chromosomal abnormalities and microdeletion syndromes through a simple maternal blood test. This innovative technology analyses cell-free fetal DNA in the mother's blood to identify potential genetic disorders, providing valuable insights for expectant parents.

For example, NIPS test can screen for:

- *Aneuploidies (abnormal number of chromosomes):* Down syndrome (Trisomy 21), Edwards syndrome (Trisomy 18), Patau syndrome (Trisomy 13), and Turner syndrome (Monosomy X).
- *Sex chromosome abnormalities:* Klinefelter syndrome (XXY), Triple X syndrome (XXX), and Jacobs syndrome (XYY).
- *Mosaicism (mix of normal and abnormal cells):* Detection of mosaicism for chromosomes 13, 18, 21, X, and Y.
- Fetal blood group assessment in Rh-negative mothers
- *Microdeletion syndromes:* Some of the microdeletion syndromes detected by NIPS are—
    - DiGeorge syndrome (22q11.2 deletion)
    - Prader-Willi syndrome (15q11.2 deletion)
    - Angelman syndrome (15q11.2 deletion)
    - Cri-du-chat syndrome (5p deletion)
    - Wolf-Hirschhorn syndrome (4p deletion)
    - Miller-Dieker syndrome (17p13.3 deletion)
    - Jacobsen syndrome (11q23 deletion)

NIPS can be performed as early as 9–10 weeks of gestation, with optimal results typically obtained between 12–22 weeks. Fetal fraction refers to the percentage of cell-free fetal DNA in the mother's blood. A higher fetal fraction increases the accuracy of NIPS results. Typically, >4% fetal fraction is desired to increase accuracy of testing.

Evidence: The American College of Obstetricians and Gynecologists (ACOG) recommends NIPS screening between 12–20 weeks. The American College of Medical Genetics and Genomics (ACMG) has issued a clinical guideline recommending non-invasive prenatal screening (NIPS) for fetal chromosome abnormalities in all pregnant individuals, regardless of risk factors. The guideline emphasizes NIPS's high accuracy and safety, and provides guidance on testing, interpretation, and counseling to ensure informed decision-making and optimal care. A systematic review of NIPS using cell-free DNA in general-risk pregnancies found that NIPS is highly accurate for detecting Trisomy 21, 18, and 13, and can be offered as a primary screening test for all pregnant women. However, the review also noted that NIPS has limitations, including a small risk of false positives and false negatives, and should be used in conjunction with ultrasound and other screening tests to ensure comprehensive fetal risk assessment. Current recommendations by the American College of Obstetricians and Gynecologists (ACOG) also states that all pregnant patients should be offered prenatal genetic screening (serum screening with or without nuchal translucency, ultrasound or cell-free DNA screening) and diagnostic testing (chorionic villus sampling CVS or amniocentesis) regardless of age or risk (Current ACOG Guidance 2024). It further reiterates the fact that cell-free DNA testing is the most accurate screening test for common genetic disorders, however, it is not a diagnostic test. In Indian clinical genetic practice, it is the obstetrician's call to judicially follow ACOG/ACMG guidelines considering the socio-economic, traditional concepts, cultural and ethnic background of pregnant women. With evolving technologies, NIPS is likely to become a standard tool for whole genome analysis and will be future for comprehensive prenatal care, empowering expectant parents with valuable information to make informed reproductive decisions.

Q2. What is the future of genome sequencing in prenatal diagnosis?

The obstetrician is soon going to face 'Fetal Genome Sequencing' as a diagnostic tool which includes exome sequencing and genome sequencing for diagnosis in both prenatal and postnatal settings. The clinician's knowledge about the phenotypic information is shown to be crucial in identifying the variant (genomic defect) as the cause of individual's symptoms. Fetal phenotypes evolve during pregnancy and fetal imaging limitations, viz., operator dependent and also fetal imaging does not detect certain subtle features. The fetal genome data analysis may give misdiagnosis due to various factors such as—incomplete fetal phenotype information by the doctor, noninclusion of gene-disease associations in published OMIM database, bioinformatics gaps or new gene-disorder discoveries. Thus, pretest genetic counseling will soon be the integral part of obstetric genetics practice as it is important to discuss with pregnant couple the reporting policies from different laboratories and parental preferences. Because variant classification in exome report can vary significantly as "Likely Pathogeneic (LP)" by one laboratory while "Variant of Unknown Significance (VUS)" by another laboratory.

The prenatal genomic diagnostics is advancing at an astonishing pace with technological improvements. The future research needs to involve a team approach consisting of basic and applied scientists, obstetricians/clinicians, parents/couples, health economists, and ethic professionals to assess the benefits and limitations of the present and new approaches. Needless to emphasize that every country might differ in their choices based on their national priorities, affordability and other health indicators. The day is not so far away to see the newborn genomic screening for early detection and prevention of genetic disorders.

Evidence: Currently, studies on fetal genome sequencing (GS) have given the evidence of only modest increase in diagnostic yield over chromosomal microarray (CMA) plus exome sequencing (ES). Future research directions therefore would be in the development of noncoding genome region analysis, powerful bioinformatics tools and the use of long-read genomic sequencing. The ability to sequence fetal genome directly from fetal tissue and indirectly from maternal blood and understanding of the fetal normal and abnormal physiology by gene expression arrays have opened up the new era of personalized medicine approach to the fetus. The future emphasis with the advanced technical capabilities will be to identify new fetal therapies with a translational approach in clinical care.

Q3. What is the impact of technology improvement in fetal ultrasonography and MRI?

The great impact of technology improvement in fetal ultrasonography (USG) and MRI in obstetric genetics cannot be denied. The last few decades have witnessed the evolution of 3D and 4D technology which is a crucial technology to predict prenatally several fetal malformations and congenital birth defects which have underlying genetic factors. The ultrasonography and MRI have definitely made a breakthrough in clinical practice of obstetric genetics, thereby helping genetic counseling to prevent the recurrence risk in the affected family.

The USG utilizes high-frequency sound waves to produce detailed images of fetal structures in a non-invasive, safe, and cost-effective manner. No doubt, it has enhanced diagnostic accuracy and patient care by providing real-time visualization and expanding its scope of applications. Traditional 2D ultrasound imaging provided flat, two-dimensional images of the fetus. In contrast, 3D ultrasound generates detailed, three-dimensional images, allowing for better visualization of fetal anatomy. The 4D ultrasound takes it a step further, providing real-time, moving images of the fetus, enabling observation of its movements and behavior.

The various genomic syndromes can thus be diagnosed on the very basis of this morphological and structural variation knowledge. The "obstetric scans" or "gene scans" play a significant role throughout pregnancy by monitoring fetal growth and allowing a unique opportunity for early interaction with the fetus. Advanced ultrasound technologies like Doppler, 3D, and 4D imaging provide detailed images of fetal anatomy thereby predicting normal or abnormal tissue/organ development which can well be correlated with genomic variants for further intervention and management. Some of the examples are as below:

- *Advanced fetal echocardiography* for the detailed examination of the fetal heart, enabling early detection of congenital heart defects which in turn can point at the specific genetic syndrome (e.g., Di-George syndrome). The timely couple genetic counseling further eases out the management and the reproductive option to the family.
- *3D neurosonography* enables the examination of the fetal brain in multiple planes, improving the detection of subtle abnormalities like corpus callosum dysgenesis, cerebellar vermis growth reduction, cortical abnormalities, etc., by accurate measurements. The incidence of congenital CNS anomalies is reported to be 83.3% on USG in suspected congenital malformations and the most common being anencephaly, holoprosencephaly, hydrocephalus, occipital encephalocele, and Dandy–Walker syndrome. The inheritance pattern and genetic implications with recurrence risk of such fetal anomalies allow sufficient time for genetic counseling and help in reproductive options or management support.

The technical advancement like spatiotemporal image correlation (STIC) facilitates the rapid acquisition of 4D volumes, reducing motion artifacts and live 4D display, allowing simultaneous examination of two orthogonal planes of the fetal heart (organ). Similarly, silhouette fetal imaging allows high-resolution 3D imaging of the fetus, creating a detailed silhouette of the fetal anatomy by detecting surface abnormalities. Likewise, virtual reality (VR) and augmented reality (AR) integration technologies enable immersive visualization of 3D/4D ultrasound data, thereby enhancing understanding of fetal anatomy to accurately guide for the interpretation of prenatal/familial genomic data. Furthermore, the abnormal USG findings contribute immensely in postnatal or prenatal intrauterine surgical planning and support genetic counseling.

In addition to genetic testing and USG, *the fetal MRI* also improves the prenatal diagnosis of many genetic disorders as it evaluates malformations. Although initial role of fetal MRI in prenatal diagnosis is limited, it does detect 90% of normal structures as per the ACOG guidelines. The structural chromosomal derangements often associated with intellectual abnormalities or yet unidentified de novo chromosomal aberrations are often difficult to predict prenatally. In such scenarios, detailed fetal MRI offers additional information which help in counseling the parents. The characteristic morphological brain abnormalities in suspected familial cases of certain inborn errors of metabolism (IEM) and correlative biochemical/enzyme deficiency together with fetal MRI findings improve the prenatal diagnosis, e.g., Tay–Sach's Disease, MPS or peroxisomal disorders or PDH (Pyruvate Lactate Deficiency).

Another example is tuberous sclerosis which is an autosomal dominant syndrome with 1 in 6,000 prevalence rate and manifests seizures, mental retardation, neurocutaneous lesions, and a variety of developmental disorders including autism. Two genes-*TSC1* on chromosome 9q34 encoding hamartin and *TSC2* gene on chromosome *16p13.3* encoding tuberin are responsible with more than 400 mutations, often de novo. The underlying lesions of Tuberous sclerosis such as cortical tubers and subependymal nodules are visualized at 21 weeks gestation indicating a good example of the combined genetic testing and fetal MRI. In the coming years with more and more new genetic disorders discovered, chromosomal and genomic DNA testing coupled with fetal MRI will become a powerful tool for prenatal diagnosis. It would then be very rational to stress the importance of research in publishing rare genotypes and their fetal MRI findings by attending obstetricians and radiologists as team members.

No doubt, the evolution of 3D, 4D ultrasound, and MRI technology has transformed the fetal genomic insights by having a supportive confirmative role in prenatal genetic diagnosis and reproductive decisions. As these technologies continue to advance, we can expect improved diagnostic accuracy, personalized prenatal care, and innovative applications that redefine the boundaries of USG and MRI imaging.

Q4. Is there a future of telemedicine in obstetric genetic healthcare?

No doubt, a telemedicine holds promising future in genetic healthcare in 21st century, especially with advances in genomic technologies. It is not only going to be efficient cost-effective tool of genetic practice, but will soon benefit the unreachable and untapped population in a cost-effective manner.

The COVID-19 pandemic has accelerated the adoption of telemedicine in obstetrics and gynecology worldwide, enabling the integration of training into remote consultations to develop essential skills. The future of telemedicine in obstetrics healthcare holds immense promise. It has already revolutionized the way expectant mothers receive prenatal care in developed countries with neither adverse effects nor unequivocal benefits.

With advancements in digital technology, telemedicine is slowly becoming an integral part of obstetric care, enabling remote monitoring, virtual consultations, and enhanced patient engagement in India. This shift, it is hoped to improve access to quality care, particularly for high-risk pregnancies, rural or underserved populations, and those with mobility issues. Telemedicine will also facilitate more frequent, shorter virtual visits, reducing the need for in-person appointments and enhancing the overall pregnancy experience. When only 2% doctors in India practice in rural areas with grossly deficient in medical facilities and infrastructure, telemedicine offers a solution to bridge the gap between available resources and growth needs in healthcare.

The primary objectives of telemedicine is to enhance the quality of healthcare, foster a virtual community of physicians, increase convenience and efficacy, and reduce medical costs. High patient's satisfaction with telemedicine can pave the way for its successful adoption and integration into routine patient care, particularly in low-resource countries where it can help to bridge healthcare gaps and improve access to quality care.

Nevertheless, there are certain pitfalls as below, majority of which are applicable to rural population which is a challenge to genetic healthcare services:

- *Technical issues:* Connectivity problems, poor video quality, and platform compatibility can hinder effective communication.
- *Limited physical examination:* Telemedicine makes it difficult to perform physical examinations, which can lead to missed diagnosis or delayed detection of genetic complications.
- *Patient's engagement and compliance:* Patients may struggle with technology or feel disconnected from their provider, leading to reduced engagement and adherence to treatment plans. Telemedicine may lack the personal touch and empathy of in-person interactions, potentially affecting patient-counselor relationships. Face-to-face communication is preferred for sensitive topics, like familial genetic condition.
- *Data privacy and security:* Telemedicine increases the risk of data breaches and cyber-attacks, compromising patient confidentiality which is of utmost importance in genetic counseling.
- *Limited access to technology:* Some patients may face barriers in accessing reliable internet, devices, or digital literacy, exacerbating health disparities. Rural patients often have limited access to technology (e.g., smartphones and computers).

The genetic healthcare should reach out to the patients and families from remote rural areas affected with common genetic conditions and who can receive benefits of the telegenetic counseling which is soon going to surpass any other clinical diagnostic testing. The empowering affected patients with education and awareness about inheritance and prevention of genetic disorders will become the future in resource-constraint countries like India. An Indian study on a role of telemedicine, an online platform "e-Sanjeevani" has concluded that teleconsultation can help to divert noncritical patients who require only medical management away from hospitals, easing the congestion at tertiary facilities and enabling more efficient allocation of resources.

As telemedicine continues to evolve, we can expect to see increased integration of artificial intelligence, machine learning, and data analytics to personalize care and predict potential genetic complications. Virtual reality and augmented reality may also be used for patient's education and prenatal care. Furthermore, telemedicine will enable seamless communication between genetic counselors and prospective patients/pregnant women, ensuring coordinated care and reducing expenses. Tele-mentoring and tele-simulation training offer opportunities for remote supervision, expert review and assessment, enhancing learning outcomes and patient care in a hybrid or fully remote setting. This could be possible in prevention and prenatal care of common hemoglobinopathies, like sickle-cell disease and thalassemia, thereby reducing the national burden of genetic disorders.

As the technology advances, telegenetic consultation is likely to become an indispensable tool in modern obstetrics with genetic implications, transforming the way we deliver prenatal care. Thus, with the rise of telegenetic counseling and digital imaging technologies, obstetric genetics will emerge as more patient-centered, effective and leading to personalized fetal care.

Q5. Will artificial intelligence (AI) play a role in future obstetric genetic care?

Yes, the artificial intelligence (AI) will definitely play a major role soon in obstetric genetic healthcare as done in other scientific disciplines. AI is a revolutionary technology that enables machines to simulate human intelligence, learning, and decision-making capabilities.

AI involves the development of algorithms and systems that can process vast amounts of data, recognize patterns, and make predictions or decisions with minimal human intervention. In the context of clinical and genomic diagnostics, AI is defined as any computer system that correctly interpret health data as observed by humans and has potential to improve diagnostic accuracy, streamline clinical/laboratory workflow and enhance patient outcome. The significance of AI is immense in obstetric genetics as it encompasses the following areas which hold tremendous research and technology update potential:

- To enhance fetal monitoring and detection of pregnancy complications in a variety of genetic conditions.
- Identify high-risk patients and predict preterm labor.
- Analyze vast genomic data emerging out of advanced next generation sequencing technology and to determine risk factors.
- To simplify and streamline pipelines of bioinformatics in genomic and fetal imaging analysis.
- Revolutionize obstetric surgery with augmented reality and 3D printing technologies.

Computer vision is an interdisciplinary field that focuses on acquiring, processing, and analyzing images and/or video. Computer vision algorithms ingest high dimensional image data and synthesize (or "convolute") it to produce numerical or symbolic representations of concepts that are embedded in the image. This process is thought to mimic the way humans identify patterns and extract meaningful features from images. Deep-learning algorithms such as Convoluted Neural Networks (CNNs) have been designed to perform computer vision tasks.

Some of the first medical imaging AI applications include the automated quantification of blood flow through the heart via cardiac MRI, the determination of ejection fraction from echocardiograms, the detection and volumetric quantification of lung nodules from radiographs, the detection and quantification of breast densities via mammography, the detection of stroke, brain bleeds, and other conditions from CT scan and automated screening for diabetic retinopathy from comprehensive dilated eye examination.

Like imaging, potential genetic disorders can be detected by speech recognition algorithms and have proved to be informative in neurological disorders like Alzheimer's and Parkinson's disease. AI and machine learning (ML) are being used in areas such as ultrasound and magnetic resonance for analysis and interpretation of images. AI-powered algorithms can be taught to precisely detect and categorize various features within these images, such as the placenta or fetal anomaly, with high degree of accuracy.

As AI continues to evolve, it is essential to address the limitations, ethical considerations, and potential biases to ensure safe and effective integration into clinical practice. By embracing AI, healthcare professionals can unlock new possibilities for improving patient's care and outcomes. The study has reported the gynecological artificial intelligence diagnostics (GAID) achieved an average accuracy of 0.85 in diagnosing patients, comparable to senior consultants by providing clear explanations for its diagnosis, fostering trust among clinicians and offered a practical database for structured history-taking assistance, patient record-keeping and expanded differential diagnosis. It is envisaged that in the future, AI will play a vital role in predicting and preventing complications during pregnancy, fetal wellbeing, childbirth, and postpartum care.

Machine learning algorithms will analyze vast amounts of data from electronic health records (EHR), medical imaging, and wearable devices to identify high-risk patients, detect early warning signs of complications, and enable personalized interventions, all of these have high genetic implication. *Artificial intelligence integration* is AI-powered automation of fetal biometry measurements which increases reliability and reproducibility, reducing scanning time and operator fatigue. AI-assisted technologies simplify fetal cardiac examinations, reduce operator dependency, and improve detection of congenital heart defects.

AI-powered diagnostic tools are useful in enhancing the accuracy and speed of disease detection, such as cervical cancer screening, ovarian cyst diagnosis, and fetal anomaly detection. The various AI-driven algorithms have already addressed many steps involved in clinical genomic analysis—including variant calling, genome annotation, variant classification and phenotype-to-genotype correlation and perhaps eventually they can also be applied for genotype-to-phenotype predictions. Thus, AI also optimizes clinical workflows, streamlining tasks, and reduces administrative burdens, allowing to focus on high value and personalized patient care. AI systems have proven to be the state-of the-art methods and have gained Food and Drug Administration (FDA) clearance for a variety of clinical diagnostics, especially imaging-based diagnostics. Currently, the most promising applications of AI in clinical genomics appear to be the AI extraction of deep phenotypic information from images, EHRs, and other medical devices to inform downstream genetic analysis. Yet, the utility of AI algorithms in predicting common complex human phenotypes has not been convincingly demonstrated.

The research studies with focus on: (1) Prenatal genomic sequencing for possible fetal abnormalities, (2) rapid genomic sequencing for critically ill children, and (3) reanalysis of genomic data obtained from children for diagnostic purposes have discussed various ethical issues in the possible application of genomic AI in these settings. These are related to concepts of beneficence, nonmaleficence, respect for autonomy, justice, transparency, accountability, privacy, and trust.

As AI continues to advance, we can expect to see more sophisticated genomic applications, such as personalized medicine, precision diagnostics, and targeted gene therapies. AI will help to unlock the secrets of the human genome, enabling tailored treatments for conditions like dysmorphic genetic syndromes, endometriosis, PCOS, and infertility. Furthermore, AI-driven research will accelerate the discovery of new treatments, vaccines, and diagnostic tools, improving health outcomes for women and babies worldwide. By embracing AI, the obstetric clinicians and molecular geneticists will experience a seismic shift in genomic era, transforming the lives of patients, care-providers, and families.

Q6. Will the robotic surgeries hold a future in obstetric genetic practice?

Surely yes! Like in case of other precision fields where robotics is helping to improve human skills and ability to the fullest, it is also going to have a great impact in obstetric genetic practice. No doubt, the technical limitations, trained manpower, finances, and ease of availability will decide the frequent utility of robotics in future patient healthcare.

The evolution of minimally invasive surgery has enabled surgeons to perform complex procedures with enhanced precision and reduced recovery time. Building on the foundation of laparoscopic hysterectomy, introduced by Harry Rich in the early 1990s, surgeons have pushed the boundaries of laparoscopic surgery, tackling increasingly complex cases. However, as surgical complexity rises, so does the risk of conversion to open surgery, particularly in patients with complex pathology and comorbidities such as higher BMI. This is where robotic-assisted surgery comes in as a game-changer introduced in 2005, utilizing computer-programmed machines to execute intricate series of actions, revolutionizing the field of surgery.

Robotic-assisted procedures offer benefits such as:

- Less pain and scarring
- Shorter recovery time
- Improved precision and dexterity
- Enhanced visualization
- Reduced blood loss

Considering the obstetric genetics, the much unexplored area is the fetal surgery for congenital birth defects which is still a distant hope! In case of a fetus diagnosed with a severe congenital anomaly, the surgery may offer an alternative to abortion, intra-uterine death, or a life with disability.

The correction of an anatomical defect reversing the associated pathophysiology in animal models was the first application of fetal surgery in the early 1980s at the California University and followed by the first successful human fetal surgical procedure in 1983 when Michael Harrison, the father of fetal surgery corrected a urinary tract congenital obstruction. Since then an improvement in fetal surgery for a number of severe fetal anomalies with regard to diagnose, select and operate have been reported in few centers worldwide, but none with success so far in India. Reduction of maternal and fetal risk are the key factors in terms of preterm labor and prematurity during fetal surgery.

Robotic-assisted procedures enable more precise and individualized care, tailoring treatments to each patient's unique needs and anatomy with more effective and minimally invasive options for patients. No doubt, it enhances the operative field's visualization, facilitating more precise and accurate procedures. The micromachines and robotic technology could step in together by providing sensory feedback and stereoscopic vision within the uterus for complex operating procedures.

The sophisticated robotic platforms enable real-time adjustment and manipulation of the surgical camera, providing surgeons with a clear and detailed view of the operative field. By optimizing visualization, these systems facilitate accurate tissue identification, precise instrument placement, and meticulous surgical technique, ultimately improving procedural efficiency and patient outcomes. For example, the closure of myelomeningocele with robotic assistance. A remotely guided device in the amniotic space with image assistance to target location for intervention procedure can be possible, viz., in case severe congenital diaphragmatic hernia to guide and deploy a reversible occlusive device within fetal trachea.

The integration of AI and machine learning algorithms has revolutionized surgical procedures by assisting in real-time decision making, surgical planning, and enhancement of robotic precision. AI algorithms can analyze vast amounts of patient's data and surgical outcomes to identify patterns and trends, enabling surgeons to make more informed decisions during procedures.

With ongoing innovations and expanding applications, robotic surgery will become a cornerstone of intrauterine fetal surgery, transforming the way surgeons treat fetus as a patient with surgical interventions. If cost issues are addressed, robotic-assisted surgery has the potential to become a popular choice among surgeons worldwide due to its technical advantages. Robotic surgery has recently advanced significantly due to minimally invasive surgical modality. It is hoped that the technological advancements will aim to overcome current limitations such as cost, extended operation time, and anesthesia time. Future research directions include developing smaller robotic equipment, remote surgery capabilities, and reducing setup and surgical time. Favorable outcomes of fetal surgeries have been reported despite existing complications. A miniaturized micro-robots are developed with the potential to eliminate or resolve the surgical complications and to further advance fetal care.

In the future, robotic-assisted surgeries will become increasingly prevalent, enabling surgeons to perform complex procedures with enhanced dexterity, visualization, and control. This will lead to reduced recovery times, less postoperative pain, and minimized scarring for patients. Robotic systems will continue to evolve, incorporating advanced technologies like artificial intelligence, machine learning, and real-time imaging, further improving surgical outcomes and expanding the range of treatable congenital birth conditions.

FUTURE DIRECTIONS

The scope for exploring many patient-related genetic issues in obstetrics and possibility of solving those with novel research approach have been elaborated individually in the above points. Incorporation of new genomic tests into current prenatal diagnosis is the need of today consisting of professional training, appropriate safety, and quality guidelines, including ethics and privacy of the affected couples/families. The detection of fetal anomaly or any abnormal function at earliest gestation period of 9–10 weeks must be targeted for successful prevention and early intervention to ensure further normal development of the unborn fetus.

Finally, the team approach of basic scientists and translational research professionals will succeed with involvement of clinicians, ethicists and affected parents/patients/family members. The personalized therapy approach to the fetus affected with genetic conditions is soon going to be the responsibility of the treating obstetrician.

BIBLIOGRAPHY

1. Agrawal P, Suman TP, Banakar S, et al. Fetal 3D Imaging and HDlive Silhouette in unraveling a rare case of gall bladder anomaly with fetal MRI correlation. J Fetal Med. 2022;9:29-33.
2. American College of Obstetricians and Gynecologists. (2024). Current ACOG Guidance. [online] Available from https://www.acog.org/advocacy/policy-priorities/non-invasive-prenatal-testing/current-acog-guidance. [Last accessed November, 2024].
3. Atkinson J, Hastie R, Walker S, et al. Telehealth in antenatal care: recent insights and advances. BMC Med. 2023;21(1):332.
4. Badeau M, Lindsay C, Blais J, et al. Genomics-based non-invasive prenatal testing for detection of fetal chromosomal aneuploidy in pregnant women. Cochrane Database Syst Rev. 2017;11(11):CD011767.
5. Bankar GR, Keoliya A. Robot-assisted surgery in gynecology. Cureus. 2022; 14(9):e29190.
6. Bianchi D. From prenatal genomic diagnosis to fetal personalized medicine: progress and challenges. Nat Med. 2012;18 (7):1041-51.
7. Coghlan S, Gyngell C, Vears DF. Ethics of artificial intelligence in prenatal and pediatric genomic medicine. J Community Genet. 2024;15(1):13-24.
8. Dias R, Torkamani A. Artificial intelligence in clinical and genomic diagnostics. Genome Med. 2019;11:70.
9. Dungan JS, Klugman S, Darilek S, et al.; ACMG Board of Directors. Noninvasive prenatal screening (NIPS) for fetal chromosome abnormalities in a general-risk population: an evidence-based clinical guideline of the American College of Medical Genetics and Genomics (ACMG). Genet Med. 2023;25(2): 100336.
10. Fahim YM, El-sharkawy MK, El-Mageed MA, et al. Role of 3D/4D Ultrasound in Assessment of Fetal Congenital Anomalies. Al-Azhar Int Med J. 2023;4:84-9.
11. Hui L, Ellis K, Mayen D, et al. Position statement from the International Society for Prenatal Diagnosis on the use of non-invasive prenatal testing for the detection of fetal chromosomal conditions in singleton pregnancies. Prenat Diagn. 2023;43(7):814-28.
12. Jayashankar SS, Nasaruddin ML, Hassan MF, et al. Non-Invasive Prenatal Testing (NIPT): Reliability, Challenges, and Future Directions. Diagnostics (Basel). 2023; 13(15):2570.

13. Kaeley N, Choudhary S, Mahala P, et al. Current scenario, future possibilities and applicability of telemedicine in hilly and remote areas in India: a review protocol. J Fam Med Prim Care. 2021;10:77-83.
14. Kiani AK, Paolacci S, Scanzano P, et al. Prenatal genetic diagnosis: Fetal therapy as a possible solution to a positive test. Acta Biomed. 2020;91(13-S):e2020021.
15. Lazier J, Hartley T, Brock JA, et al. Clinical application of fetal genome-wide sequencing during pregnancy: position statement of the Canadian College of Medical Geneticists. J Med Genetics. 2022;59:931-7
16. Magann EF, McKelvey SS, Hitt WC, et al. The use of telemedicine in obstetrics: a review of the literature. Obstet Gynecol Surv. 2011;66(3):170-8.
17. Manickam K, McClain M, Demmer LA, et al. Exome and genome sequencing for pediatric patients with congenital anomalies or intellectual disability: an evidence-based clinical guideline of the American College of Medical Genetics and Genomics (ACMG). Genet Med. 2021;23:2029-37.
18. Mohapatra I, Rai VK, Samantaray SR. Impact of telemedicine on antenatal care at a teaching institution in Eastern India: an insight into the future of better India. J Fam Med Prim Care. 2023;12(11):2652-60.
19. Nobbenhuis MAE, Gul N, Barton-Smith P, et al. Robotic surgery in gynaecology: Scientific Impact Paper No. 71 (July 2022). BJOG. 2023;130(1):e1-e8.
20. Nogué L, Gómez O, Izquierdo N, et al. Feasibility of 4D-Spatio Temporal Image Correlation (STIC) in the Comprehensive Assessment of the Fetal Heart Using FetalHQ®. J Clin Med. 2022;11(5):1414.
21. Park J, Bak S, Song JY, et al. Robotic surgery in gynecology: the present and the future. Obstet Gynecol Sci. 2023;66(6):518-28.
22. Recker F, Gembruch U, Strizek B. Clinical Ultrasound Applications in Obstetrics and Gynecology in the Year 2024. J Clin Med. 2024;13(5):1244.
23. Rose NC, Barrie ES, Malinowski J, et al; ACMG Professional Practice and Guidelines Committee. Systematic evidence-based review: the application of noninvasive prenatal screening using cell-free DNA in general-risk pregnancies. Genet Med. 2022;24(7):1379-91.
24. Singh A, Agarwal A, Thakur G, et al. Role of telemedicine in obstetrics and gynecology: an experience at tertiary care center. Expert Rev Med Devices. 2023;20(12):1251-6.
25. Tanos P, Yiangou I, Prokopiou G, et al. Gynaecological Artificial Intelligence Diagnostics (GAID) GAID and Its Performance as a Tool for the Specialist Doctor. Healthcare. 2024;12(2):223.
26. Ushakov F, Sacco A, Pandya P. First-trimester 3D fetal neurosonography: five standardised views. J Obstet Gynaecol. 2024;44(1):2361848.
27. Wang L, Nie H, Wang Q, et al. Use of magnetic resonance imaging combined with gene analysis for the diagnosis of fetal congenital heart disease. BMC Med Imaging. 2019;19(1):12.
28. Wojcik MH, Reimers R, Poorvu T, et al. Genetic diagnosis in the fetus. J Perinatol. 2020;40(7):997-1006.
29. Yadav P, Chaudhari K, Dave A, et al. Exploring the evolution of robotic surgery in obstetrics and gynecology: past, present, and future perspectives. Cureus. 2024;16(3):e57155.
30. Yazdani A, Costa S, Kroon B. Artificial intelligence: Friend or foe? Aust N Z J Obstet Gynaecol. 2023;63:127-30.